HOPE IN HELL
INSIDE THE WORLD OF DOCTORS WITHOUT BORDERS

DAN BORTOLOTTI

FIREFLY BOOKS

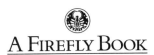

A FIREFLY BOOK

Published by Firefly Books Ltd. 2006

First printing

Publisher Cataloging-in-Publication Data   (U.S.)

Bortolotti, Dan.

  Hope in hell : inside the world of Doctors without Borders / Dan Bortolotti. — Rev. ed.

[304] p. : photos. (some col.) ;   cm.
Includes bibliographical references and index.

Summary: Account of the experiences of individual medical professionals who work for Doctors without Borders around the world, including Africa, Asia and Europe. Covers how Doctors without Borders was founded and how the organization has reacted to recent world events.

ISBN-13: 978-155407-142-5
ISBN-10: 1-55407-142-9 (pbk.)

  1. Doctors without Borders (Association). 2. Physicians. 3. Disaster medicine. I. Title.

610/.6/01 dc22   RA390.F8B67 2005

Library and Archives Canada Cataloguing in Publication

Bortolotti, Dan

  Hope in hell : inside the the world of Doctors Without Borders / Dan Bortolotti. — Rev. ed.

Includes bibliographical references and index.

ISBN-13: 978-155407-142-5
ISBN-10: 1-55407-142-9

  1. Doctors Without Borders (Association). 2. Disaster medicine. 3. War relief. I. Title.

RA390.A2B67 2006   610'.6'01   C2005-904557-4

Published in the United States by
Firefly Books (U.S.) Inc.
P.O. Box 1338, Ellicott Station
Buffalo, New York 14205

Published in Canada by
Firefly Books Ltd.
66 Leek Crescent
Richmond Hill, Ontario L4B 1H1

Cover and interior design by Sari Naworynski

Printed and bound in Canada

The publisher gratefully acknowledges the financial support for our publishing program by the Government of Canada through the Book Publishing Industry Development Program.

In memory of Penny Argue,
whose life showed that medicine has limits,
while bravery does not.

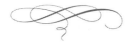

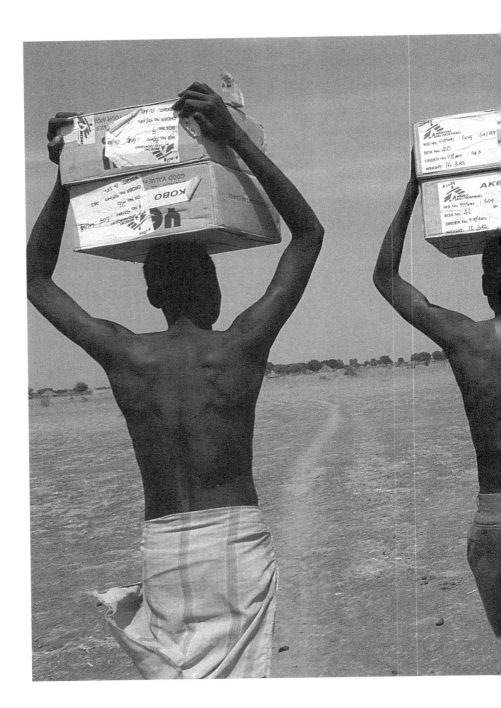

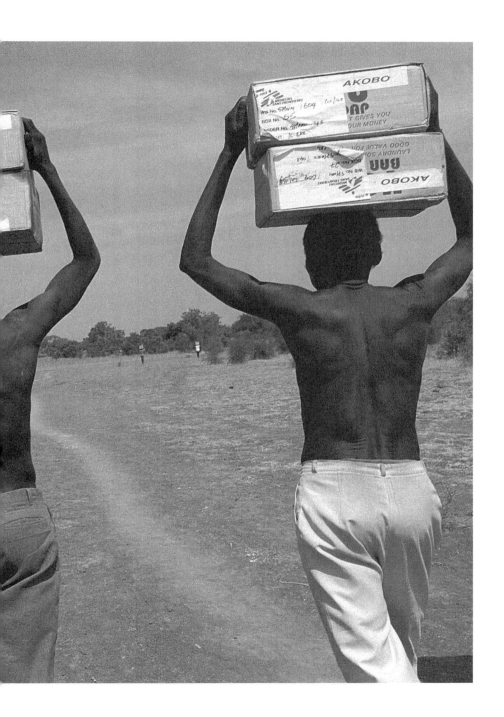

Contents

Introduction | Fixing Up the Humans

They are not Gods
though they would like to be;
they are only a human
trying to fix up a human.

— ANNE SEXTON, "DOCTORS"

Like many organizations that began modestly and grew to impressive stature, Médecins Sans Frontières has its own creation myth. The story is based in historical fact, but it's related and remembered differently by the people who were there. In the standard version, a group of young French doctors goes to work in a Red Cross hospital in the breakaway Nigerian state of Biafra in 1968. They are appalled by what they see – hundreds of thousands of children dying from malnutrition – and believe they are witnesses to a genocide. Although the Red Cross requires the utmost discretion from its volunteers, the French doctors, led by the charismatic Bernard Kouchner, cannot remain silent. They angrily tear their Red Cross armbands from their sleeves and denounce the Nigerian government. On returning to France, they organize a committee to raise awareness of the genocide and, later, a group of doctors devoted to emergency medical aid. Around the same time, a Paris medical journal publishes a call for volunteer doctors to help the victims of earthquakes and floods. The two groups eventually come together in 1971 to form Médecins Sans Frontières. More than 30 years later, journalist David Rieff, who has covered wars and emergencies around the globe, calls this group "the most important humanitarian NGO in the world."

Médecins Sans Frontières – also known in North America as Doctors Without Borders, and universally as MSF – is the world's largest independent medical humanitarian organization. Every year it sends more than 3,000 volunteers to some 80 different countries. Its most-noticed projects are in conflict zones, refugee camps and countries hit by famine, though MSF also runs smaller programs outside the media spotlight – supporting rural health clinics, providing antiretroviral treatment for people with AIDS, bringing fresh water and sanitation to remote villages.

In the expanding universe of aid agencies, where does MSF fit? To begin with, the aid community makes a clear distinction between development and relief. To borrow an old adage, relief agencies give a man a fish and feed him for a day, while development aims to teach that man to fish so he can feed himself for life. MSF has always been a relief agency, providing aid to populations in acute crisis. It almost invariably works closely with health ministries and trains local staff, and may work in an area for several years, though it does not attempt to address the underlying causes of the emergencies. MSF operates feeding centers, but does not supply shovels and seeds to grow crops; it brings health care to poor areas, but does not try to eradicate poverty.

There is also a fundamental difference between humanitarian and human rights organizations. Both uphold international law (whether the Geneva Conventions or the Universal Declaration of Human Rights), but human rights organizations tend to be more activist, with lobbying at the heart of their work. Humanitarian agencies, in contrast, remain neutral in order to get access to victims on all sides. MSF is a humanitarian organization – neutrality is enshrined in its charter – but from its earliest days it has wrestled with the knowledge that, in cases of brutality and oppression, neutrality may be tantamount to complicity.

When MSF emerged in France in 1971, nothing like it had existed before. There were other aid agencies, of course – Save the Children was already more than 50 years old, Oxfam almost 30 – but the International Committee of the Red Cross was the only group bringing significant medical relief to the victims of wars and natural disasters around the world. Now, as conflicts in the late 1970s displaced millions of people, a new private organization found a niche in the refugee camps of Southeast Asia, Africa, and Central and South America.

From the beginning, MSF's reputation exceeded its actual impact in the countries where it worked. Its early emergency projects were small, often poorly coordinated and modest in their success. Yet with the flamboyant and media-savvy Kouchner at the helm, MSF gained a reputation for going where other aid agencies would not go. Newspapers carried pictures of the fearless and heroic doctors riding into Soviet-occupied Afghanistan on donkeys, trekking the jungles of a newly independent Angola, and tending to Cambodians in the shadow of the Khmer Rouge. Among the French press and the public, Médecins Sans Frontières became known as medical mavericks, the cowboys of emergency aid, a reputation that clings to it – for better or worse – to the present day.

Inside the organization, however, tensions were simmering between the original Biafran clan and a younger generation of doctors that was growing weary of Kouchner's media stunts. In late 1978, as thousands of boat people fled Vietnam, Kouchner announced a plan to send a rescue ship (and television crews) to the China Sea, an operation most of the younger MSFers felt was naïve and futile. The arguments became bitter, and within a few months Kouchner and his allies were gone, forced out of the organization they had helped to found.

During the 1980s, MSF added offices in Belgium, Switzerland, Holland, Spain and Luxembourg – each with considerable autonomy. Its reputation continued to grow, and so did its outspokenness – MSF criticized Pol Pot's regime in Cambodia in 1980, then was expelled from Ethiopia after it did the same to Colonel Mengistu. Now well funded by UN agencies, European governments and private donors, it soon became admired for its logistics and its frugal use of resources. As its teams moved quickly and efficiently by plane, Land Cruiser, canoe and on foot to deliver medical aid to the most dangerous and remote places on earth, MSF acquired a paradoxical image. It was an informal *mouvement* with a culture of debate that nonetheless acted decisively, an organization of swashbucklers with technical expertise that spoke with equal parts brazenness and sophistication.

The 1980s has been called the golden age of humanitarianism. Western governments had not yet co-opted humanitarian aid as a tool to "win the hearts and minds" of people in occupied countries. The Ethiopian famine that began in 1983 sparked Live Aid and countless other fundraisers, and money poured into the coffers of aid agencies. Being an aid worker carried cachet, and by the end of the decade, when French citizens were surveyed about their ideal job, a third of them said they wanted to be a *médecin sans frontières*.

During the 1990s, MSF became a global organization, adding sections in the United States, Canada, Japan, Hong Kong and Australia. But as it did so, the golden age of humanitarianism gave way to an unprecedented period of soul-searching in the aid community. People shed their innocence about the impact of aid, realizing that it can create a culture of dependency and even exacerbate conflicts. The crises of those years dramatically revealed the moral ambiguity of relief and intervention – in Bosnia, where UN peacekeepers failed to stop the massacre of 7,000 people in Srebrenica; in Rwanda, where aid poured in to help Hutus who had just perpetrated the worst genocide since World War II; and in Kosovo, where the perverse term "humanitarian bombing" was born in 1999. That same year, Médecins Sans Frontières received one of the world's highest honors, the Nobel Prize for Peace.

Throughout the Cold War and the post–September 11 "war on terror," whatever style of aid happens to be popular with Western governments, MSF's doctors, nurses and other volunteers continue to grip the imagination of the public. People are captivated by the drama of surgery in war zones, the image of prosperous professionals who leave behind comfortable lives. "Without Borders" suggests a gatecrashing fearlessness that appeals to those who are tired of the timidity of the United Nations, and perhaps even the neutrality of the Red Cross.

But is that what MSF is really about? The group runs several hundred projects a year, and most are not on the front lines of conflict. The medical teams may simply train locals rather than treat patients, and most of the volunteers are not sacrificing lucrative medical careers – three-quarters are not even doctors. That's not to say that the truth is more mundane, only that it's more complex – and thankfully so. A nuanced portrait is always more interesting than a caricature.

1 | Under the Angolan Sun

Dr. James Knox slings his medical kit across his back and begins the 10-minute walk to the tiny health center in Cuimba. Along the main road in this northern Angolan village, children playing in front of adobe houses greet him with cries of *Mundele!* – the Kikongo word for white person.

Just past the market, the health center comes into view on the left. When the electricity is working, the 10 or so beds of the inpatient ward are illuminated by a solitary light bulb. Today they're lit only by the afternoon sun, which enters, along with the flies and malaria-toting mosquitoes, through the ward's two glassless windows. A mild breeze struggles heroically to vanquish the smell of unwashed bodies. Knox sits down on an empty bed to get a closer look at a newborn baby who was admitted for malnutrition a few days earlier. The mother, who can't be older than 18, was having difficulty breastfeeding, so she walked for two days from the town of Serra da Kanda, more than 30 miles to the southeast. She

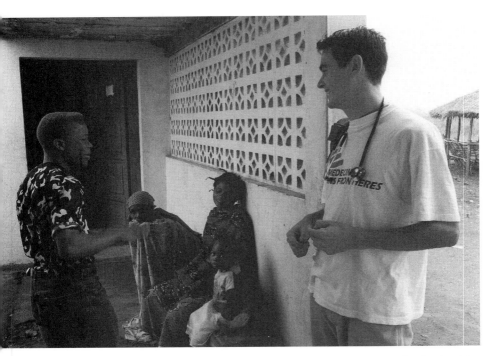

Australian physician James Knox chats with a nurse outside the health center in Cuimba, Angola. As in many MSF projects, the expat doctor's main role is to support and train local medical staff. Patients walk or bicycle from miles away, and the most seriously ill face a three-hour drive to the nearest hospital.

looks relieved as the doctor explains in Portuguese that the baby is gaining weight and is now out of danger.

Tall and slender, with black hair and expressive eyes, the 28-year-old physician says it's hard to know just what he'd be doing had he decided to practice in his native Australia – he'd probably be holding down a junior hospital position. Here, weeks into his first mission with Médecins Sans Frontières, he's the only show in town. As a volunteer, Knox will spend nine months giving health care to the 25,000 people who are

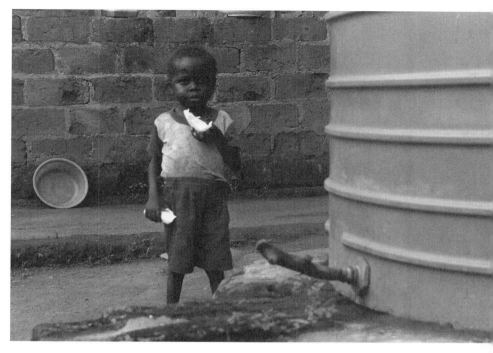

A young boy munches a high-energy BP-5 biscuit at the Cuimba health center. Recently returned from the Democratic Republic of Congo, where they had fled during Angola's decades-long war, the boy and his sister were admitted to the health center with moderate malnutrition.

expected to pass through Cuimba on their way home from the Democratic Republic of Congo. During the most recent outbreak of war, 70,000 Angolans fled to DRC – the border is just 18 miles to the north – but now that peace has endured for more than a year, many of these refugees are trickling back and trying to rebuild their lives.

As he makes his rounds, Knox is watched by a brother and sister, perhaps 4 and 5 years old, who smile at him while they munch BP-5 biscuits, high-energy supplements given to moderately malnourished children. These kids, their father explains, have just returned from DRC and have found that good food is scarce. The children have been subsisting mainly on *funge,* a gelatinous porridge made from cassava flour. It fills the belly but is devoid of protein.

When the little girl arrived she also had a fever, a red flag for malaria, which is rampant in Cuimba. With the closest lab a three-hour drive away, Knox has to rely on a rapid blood test called Paracheck. The test isn't 100 percent effective, so when it turned out negative he chose to treat her for malaria anyway. It's not the kind of decision he would have had to make at home. In a Western hospital, diagnosis is often made with a battery of sophisticated instruments. Here, the technology at Knox's disposal fits into his shoulder bag: stethoscope, blood pressure cuff, thermometer, otoscope and a copy of MSF's *Essential Drugs* manual. There's also the language barrier to contend with. Knox can handle the Portuguese, but many of those returning from the Congo speak only French or Kikongo. "Sometimes the patient histories, when they're translated into Portuguese, are not all that reliable. You have to depend more on the physical signs, so you need to be a lot more observant. It really does change the way you diagnose."

Late in the afternoon, a young man arrives with his gravely ill sister after a bicycle journey of more than 40 miles. Johanna, 27, is lethargic and emaciated. Her brother says she's had a cough for about two weeks, but after his examination Knox suspects she's been sick for much longer. Her hipbones protrude sharply, her ribcage is clearly visible, her skin barely springs back when pinched. When a nurse asks her to sit up, she vomits. Knox gets her started on oral rehydration salts, but he fears that dehydration is only the beginning of her problems. "It looks like sleeping sickness," he says.

Several old women shuffle around outside the ward, one wearing a T-shirt improbably emblazoned with the words *Extreme Hockey*. It's late in the afternoon now, and while the temperature is still well over 70 degrees Fahrenheit, two of them ask for blankets and perhaps a bit of food. But the health center has nothing to spare.

You have to go back a long way to find peace in Angola. The first Portuguese missionaries arrived in this large southwest African country – almost twice the size of Texas – in the 1490s. Some 35 miles west of Cuimba in Mbanza Congo, capital of the old kingdom of Kongo, you can look out the window of the MSF house and still see ruins on the site of the southern hemisphere's first Catholic church. Pope John Paul II said mass there in 1992, and no one has yet bothered to dismantle the stage.

It wasn't until the mid-20th century that the Portuguese settled Angola in significant numbers, and popular uprisings began almost immediately. Portugal's dictatorship was overthrown in 1974, and colonial rule ended in Angola soon after, though fighting continued among three separate independence movements. The two that endured did so with outside help: UNITA, backed by South Africa and the United States, and the MPLA, supported by the Soviet Union and Cuba. In November 1975, the MPLA declared itself the governing party of an independent People's Republic of Angola. Throughout the 1980s, Angola – rich in oil, diamonds and coffee – was a Cold War battleground, with the UNITA rebels, led by the charismatic warrior Jonas Savimbi, pitted against the one-party socialist state of José Eduardo dos Santos.

In 1991, the MPLA and UNITA agreed to peace, and elections followed the next year. Under the watchful eye of the United States, the Soviet Union and Portugal, the presidential voting was deemed free and fair: dos Santos won 129 seats in the National Assembly to Savimbi's 70. UNITA refused to accept defeat, however, and fighting broke out almost immediately. In the brutal months that followed, most of the conflict took place in the cities, forcing thousands of people to flee as UNITA captured at least two-thirds of the country. Between 1975 and 1994, perhaps a million and a half Angolans died in the fighting or from starvation and disease, its direct consequences. When Savimbi began to lose ground in 1994, he agreed to another peace accord, brokered by South African president Nelson Mandela and signed in Lusaka, Zambia, in November. Both sides made concessions, agreeing to demobilize their troops and create a coalition government. But skirmishes resumed in 1997, followed by all-out war the following year.

During this period of the fighting – from 1998 to 2002 – human suffering in Angola reached its peak, as civilians were specifically targeted by both sides. Soldiers rounded up entire villages and used people as human shields and forced laborers – their clothing stolen so they wouldn't escape – mercilessly whipping them for disobedience. Women were raped, and their children were forced to serve as soldiers. People fled into the bush for months on end, living off of leaves, roots and maybe some honey. Though it had small projects in several parts of Angola, MSF learned the full story only later, because by 1998 humanitarian organizations were unable to work in UNITA-controlled areas – some 80 percent of the country, including Cuimba.

Finally, in February 2002, Savimbi was killed and, by April, war-weary UNITA forces and the dos Santos government agreed to another ceasefire. So far, this one has held. One of the first aid agencies to be allowed back in March of that year, MSF explored the previously inaccessible areas. What it found was appalling – the most serious malnutrition on the continent in a decade. MSF quickly set up 44 feeding centers capable of treating 14,000 malnourished children and, by the end of the year, it was more active in Angola than in any other country. Not everyone was moving so quickly, though. In June, Morten Rostrup, who was then MSF's International Council president, blasted the United Nations for its "shamefully slow and shockingly insufficient" efforts to respond to the hunger. The UN fought back, arguing that "MSF is quick to criticise but they should do more to coordinate with partners." It was just the latest example of the two organizations clashing in public. There would be more.

Cuimba is in the northwestern province of Zaire (not be confused with the former name of the Democratic Republic of Congo, which it borders), where malnutrition is less severe than in many other regions. The MSF project here is administered by an office in Holland and coordinated by teams in Luanda, the Angolan capital, and in Mbanza Congo, the provincial capital. These teams also support other projects in the region – for example, MSF has immunized the children for measles and is engaged in "active case finding" for sleeping sickness. Rather than waiting for patients to show up at the health center, MSF sends trained staff into the community to look for the deadly parasitic disease.

The organization's main activity in Cuimba is supporting the health center. Working with the local ministry of health, MSF supplies drugs and equipment, transports seriously ill patients to the hospital in Mbanza Congo, and trains the all-male nursing team. Though he examines some patients himself, James Knox spends the bulk of his time supervising the work of the local nurses and giving informal presentations in the *jangu* – a gazebo-style shelter outside the hospital, skillfully built from sticks and thatch. He knows MSF can't change things overnight, but he's doing his best to make sure the clinic follows some minimum standards. "It's difficult," he says, "because there are few nurses who even have an idea of what infection control is. When we got here, there was no place for me to wash my hands. I had to go out to the pump in front of the health center. And there was no way to dispose of sharps – they were just going into the rubbish bin with everything else. We heard that, before our arrival, needles were sometimes reused on the same patient."

MSF has dug a disposal area behind the health center where sharps are destroyed before they become children's playthings. Knox has a mental list of other priorities. "There are so many things we're trying to change that, at this early stage, I don't insist on everything," he says. "The nursing staff are not MSF employees, so if we were to make a fuss about everything all at once it would probably be counterproductive. At the moment, I insist that the nurses give the correct dose of the correct drug, in a way that is safe for the patient. I don't yet insist they wear gloves for all procedures. That will come later."

Relations with the local medical staff can make or break a project. Knox is exceptionally good at building trust, especially for someone on his first mission. He's laid-back, soft-spoken and patient in situations where Job would have been driven to madness. He respects the power structure at the health center and goes through the head of nursing, whom he affectionately addresses as *Chefe* (Boss), when he tries to make changes. He recognizes that the nurses are doing the best they can with paltry resources. One of the finest among them isn't even getting paid. If the nurses are having difficulty with a procedure, he resists the urge to jump in and do it himself. "That's not a directive I've been given," he explains, "but it just seems like the right thing to do. When I started here, I was told that I might be the only doctor who ever works in this project. And I was told that MSF has to be ready to pull out at any time."

Not all of MSF's work is in active emergencies – in addition to war zones and refugee camps, it also works in peaceful but remote corners of the world, where people have no other access to health care. Often teams will come and go for years, but that's not by design. Once the epidemic has passed, or the government has been prodded into caring for its people, or the work has been handed over to another aid agency, it's time for MSF to pull out. "But," says Knox, "to an extent you do want to leave something behind."

Sipping a warm beer outside the rented MSF staff house in June 2003, James Knox reflects on his first mission. Like most doctors who volunteer with the organization, he knows that some people look on his work as heroic, as though he had selflessly sacrificed his career and put his life on the line to help the poor and suffering. The reality is hardly that simple. "There probably are people who do this for purely altruistic reasons," he says, "but I haven't found one yet. I mean, you're helping people, but it's not exactly altruistic if there's something in it for you as well."

Admittedly, delivering humanitarian aid can be dangerous in Angola. MSF has a few rules that suggest there are potential risks, even in peacetime Cuimba: no overnight stays without a vehicle and driver on standby; no walking alone in the village after dark; always carry $50 "security money" in case of extortion or kidnapping. Everyone also gets mine-awareness training: if you're driving, follow the tracks of other vehicles and never leave the main road; if you must stop to relieve yourself during a long drive, do so behind the car.

Of course, following these security rules is hardly a guarantee. On November 29, 2002, two MSF vehicles were traveling from Cunjamba to Mavinga in southeastern Angola, returning from a small village where the occupants had spent the day giving measles vaccinations. They had driven the same road that morning, but this time the back wheel of the first Land Cruiser, jam-packed with 13 people, hit an anti-tank mine. Seven were killed – four Angolan MSF staffers, two ministry of health employees, and a baby boy.

The dangers of road travel in Angola can be even more unpredictable. MSF's policy in most African countries is clear: if you hit a person or an animal with a vehicle, you keep driving, returning only after you've notified the authorities. You don't stop to help, even if you're a doctor. It sounds coldhearted, but an incident on March 9, 2003, showed why it's necessary. Rachel Stow, a British physician working in MSF's project in Malange, was returning from Luanda with driver Aderito Augusto and an assistant when the vehicle struck and killed a young girl. When they stopped, a mob dragged Augusto from the driver's seat and brutally beat him to death. Stow narrowly managed to escape in the Land Cruiser while the assistant fled on foot.

As Knox speaks, a full moon high in the southeast casts its sheen on the sleepy village, and it's easy to feel far removed from these horror stories. Despite the potential danger, MSFers will tell you that working in a place like this is a rare privilege, particularly for a doctor who hasn't yet turned 30. Knox studied medicine in New South Wales, then took a three-month course in tropical medicine in Liverpool, England. After being accepted by MSF, he learned he would be doing his first mission in Angola, so he took a crash course in Portuguese. A few months later he was in Cuimba with just one other expat (as expatriate volunteers are known), American nurse Martha Anderson, who this week is away in Mbanza Congo. Knox and Anderson have a small but comfortable house made from sun-baked bricks. André, the project's logistician, built much of it himself, and he lives nearby with his family. Pedro, one of the drivers, also stays here when he's away from his home in Mbanza.

One of the biggest misconceptions about MSF is that the organization is primarily doctors. In fact, only about a quarter of the volunteers in the field (to say nothing of those who staff its international offices) are physicians, and more than 40 percent are nonmedical staff, including project coordinators, financial coordinators, logisticians and administrators. Although expats are the ones who attract the interest – and the donations – from the Western public, the work in the field is done mostly by locally hired medical and nonmedical staff like André and Pedro. In 2002, MSF had almost 15,000 national staff in its projects, compared with fewer than 3,000 expats.

The Cuimba house has electricity for only a few hours each night, so Knox and Anderson charge portable solar-powered lights during the day – useful for late-night trips to the outhouse, which is equipped with a standard MSF-issue squat plate. Entertainment is simple – paperback novels, a few CDs. Both have brought their guitars, and in a pinch André can scare up a drum from the local church. The beer is warm, but the one guy in town with a generator will sell you a cold can for an extra 10 kwanzaas, about 18 cents.

There's no running water, so the staff trucks in plastic barrels filled at the local pumps, then boils and filters it for drinking. Knox says he finds the cold bucket showers invigorating in the morning, and the cockroaches don't really bother him. "It's the spiders I hate," he says. A young woman from the village arrives each morning with her toddler son slung across her back. She does the laundry – mostly khakis and MSF T-shirts – makes the meals and cleans the house. Before she heads home, she leaves dinner in a pot so the doctor or nurse can heat it up on a kerosene stove. And that contraption looks more dangerous than any landmine.

Food is a source of some amusement. If you're willing to eat local delicacies, there's little problem. But if you're tired of *funge* and *kizaka*, a dish made from cassava leaves, the cook will prepare Western-style food with the available ingredients and no experience. You get spaghetti chopped into one-inch pieces, flatbread piled with vegetables in a vaguely pizza-like way, mashed potatoes topped with fried eggs and other dubious combinations. Some MSFers claim they've copped the odd BP-5 biscuit in desperation. Knox's colleagues joke that he's becoming too thin, though he insists he's lost "only a few kilos."

Next day at the Cuimba health center, James Knox asks one of the nurses about an empty bed in the back of the inpatient ward. It had been occupied by a man with an abscessed liver, but now he's gone. The nurse says he's checked himself out, and Knox gives a resigned smile. "It's frustrating," he says, "because sometimes you order a drug, and just when it arrives the patient has left. There's no way of tracking these people down." Another patient, admitted the day before for hypertension, has also vanished.

Knox wonders aloud if there's a connection between the self-discharges and an event that happened two days earlier, when he left Cuimba to travel to the better-equipped hospital in Mbanza Congo with a baby who was critically ill with malaria. "After the transfer, I noticed a change when we came back," he says. "Some of the patients were leaving before their treatment was up, and we had very few patients on the ward." Before prepping the baby for the transfer, Knox had to explain the situation to the family. "I felt obliged to inform the parents that the child might not survive, and we had to do that on the ward – because of the constraints in the health center, there really isn't very much privacy. So the rest of the ward heard this information." As it happened, the baby died later that night in Mbanza Congo. "I'm not sure how it's perceived when a white doctor says to a family, 'Your child may not survive,' and then the child is transferred and, in fact, doesn't survive."

Understanding local attitudes about illness is part of the learning curve for all expat doctors and nurses. In Cuimba, and in most places where health care is a novelty, patients often arrive only after they've become terribly ill. One man in the ward says he's been feeling pain and numbness in his arms for two months. The doctor's examination reveals some sort of mass in his abdomen, but the man insists he's ill because a family member recently gave him a poisoned drink. Sometimes the patient's condition has been worsened by traditional healers – the market, where all manner of suspect pharmaceuticals are sold, from shiny minerals to seashells to dead mice, is only a short distance from the health center.

Even the ministry of health's standard treatments, or protocols, are a challenge to overcome. The first-line drug for malaria in much of Africa is still choloroquine, but in Angola it's ineffective for up to 83 percent of patients. Part of MSF's goal here, and in every other antimalarial program it runs, is to implement a far more effective treatment called artemisinin-based combination therapy. Knox and Anderson know first-hand how well it works – they're both just getting over malaria themselves, an occupational hazard.

Knox approaches the nurses who are examining Johanna, the young woman he suspected of having sleeping sickness. They've managed to get a little more of the patient's history, which now includes not only coughing but vomiting and lack of appetite. "It's starting to look more like TB," the doctor says. Tuberculosis is ideally confirmed with a chest x-ray, but here they can use only a sputum smear, and even that involves a transfer to Mbanza Congo.

Now another baby has arrived with signs of malaria, and a Paracheck comes up positive. As the nurses prepare an infusion of quinine, Knox notices that the bottle contains far more medication than necessary – the nurses are planning to stop the drip once the right amount is delivered and then use the same bottle for the next dose. Knox has to insist they find a clean, empty bottle in which to put the excess – otherwise, if no one remembers to check it at the right time, the child could receive an overdose.

The baby shrieks as the IV needle is inserted, and then removed when the nurse sees he's missed the vein. Three or four more attempts are unsuccessful – not surprisingly, since this procedure is difficult with a baby at the best of times, and it's harder if the patient is dehydrated. The baby's mother sits off to the side in silence, but she's clearly distressed at watching her child suffer. After a few minutes, she walks out of the ward. Knox stands by and calmly offers advice, refusing to take over from the nurses and undermine their training. It takes half an hour to get the line in place.

Then, with the drip finally established, one of the nurses picks up the IV stand and attempts to move it to the other side of the bed. In the process, he yanks the needle out of the baby's arm and they have to start over again. At one point, five nurses are working on the baby, who by this time is as stoical as the good doctor. Soon the needle is in place again, but hours later the child's arm has filled with fluid – the needle wasn't in a vein after all.

Early the next day, Knox decides to transfer another sick baby, along with Johanna, to the hospital in Mbanza Congo. He'll make the trip, too. It's only about 40 miles, but the drive takes three hours as the Land Cruiser negotiates enormous ruts and water-filled craters, challenging the passengers to keep their heads from smashing against the roof. At one point the driver struggles for a minute or two in mud that must be a couple of feet deep – and this is the dry season. Later on, the vehicle passes the carcasses of a blue pickup truck and a burned-out tank, both reminders that this road used to be mined.

Inside the car, Johanna, wearing a mask to protect the others and accompanied by a female relative, lies across one of the bench seats. The baby, in the arms of her father, looks ashen and occasionally gasps for breath. Knox gestures for a cup of water, which they try to get into the baby's mouth. She quickly spits up. Few words are exchanged during the trip, even between the Kikongo speakers, but at least no one vomits. In areas where people are unused to traveling like this, patients are often violently carsick. Last week, Anderson did this same ride with a woman who threw up repeatedly.

It's mid-afternoon when the car pulls up at the municipal hospital in Mbanza Congo. The baby and her parents quickly disappear inside as the staff carries in Johanna. Nearby, a smiling young man rides a specially designed tricycle that he pedals with his hands – his legs, withered by polio, hang limply from the seat.

Knox will return the following morning to check on the new arrivals, but then it's back to Cuimba, where he's needed more. The doctors in Mbanza Congo will take over the care of his patients, and following up isn't always possible. He never does learn their fate.

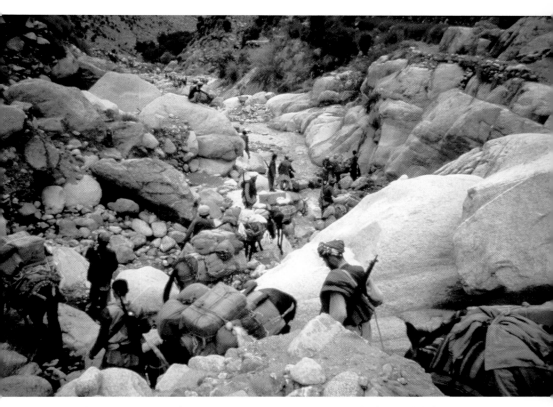

Afghan resistance fighters carry MSF supplies through the Badakshan valley in 1984. During the Soviet occupation of Afghanistan, MSF gained a reputation for delivering aid in places where no other agency would go.

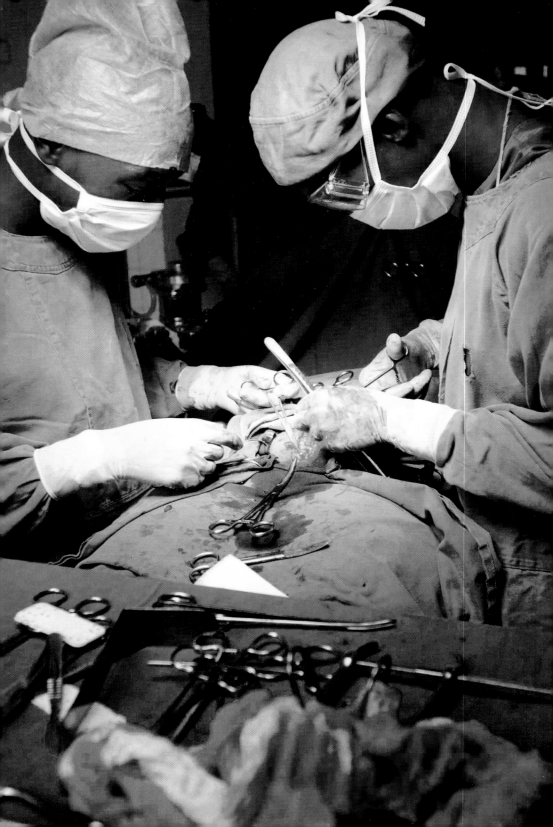

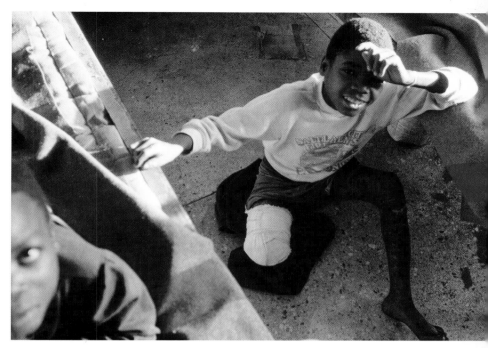

Above: A 12-year-old landmine victim recuperates in a Kuito hospital that was rehabilitated by MSF. Although Angola's civil war ended in 2002, millions of mines continue to kill and maim.

Right: A security guard peers through the door of the MSF living quarters in Monrovia in July 2003. Even in the most volatile war zones, humanitarian aid workers do not allow weapons in their vehicles or compounds.

Opposite: Surgeons attempt to save the life of an injured soldier in Bouake, Ivory Coast, in January 2003. The Bouake hospital was so overwhelmed with patients that one doctor remarked, "Darwin was part of our triage."

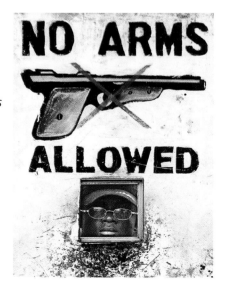

NO ARMS ALLOWED

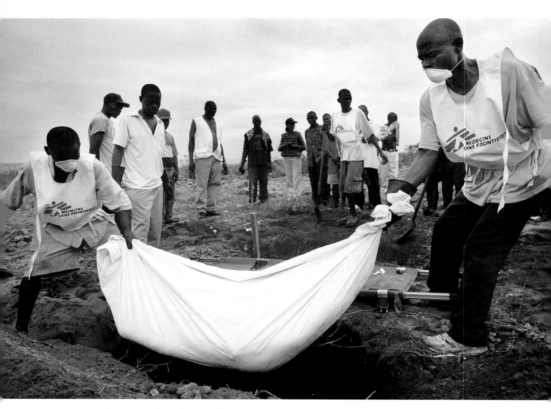

Local MSF workers bury a body in Monrovia, Liberia's capital, following an attack by rebels in July 2003. While expats have an evacuation plan in case of heavy fighting, national staff must remain behind.

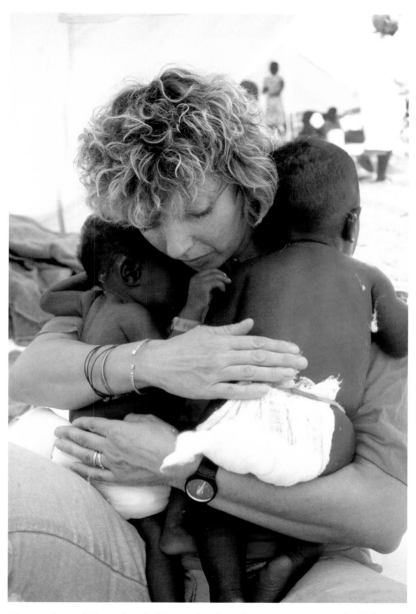

*Two orphaned Rwandan babies get a hug from an MSF expat in Zaire.
While children were not spared during the 1994 genocide, about
100,000 who lost their parents managed to escape with their own lives.*

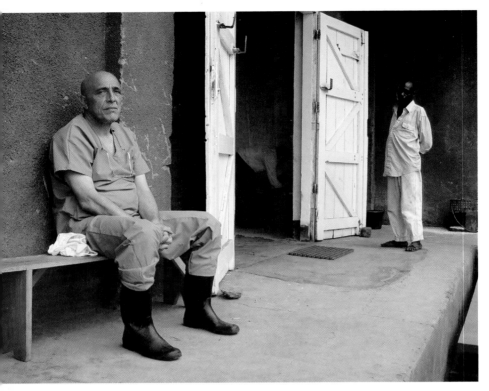

An exhausted doctor takes a break outside MSF's field hospital in Bunia, in eastern Democratic Republic of Congo, in June 2003. Conflict in the country has kept the organization active there since 1981.

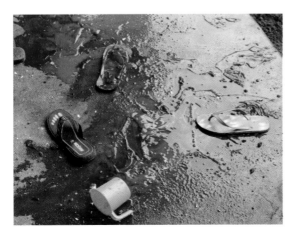

Fleeing civilians left a trail of blood and discarded items after rebels bombed Mamba Point, Liberia, in July 2003. MSF missions during Liberia's civil war of 2002 and 2003 were among the most dangerous of the period.

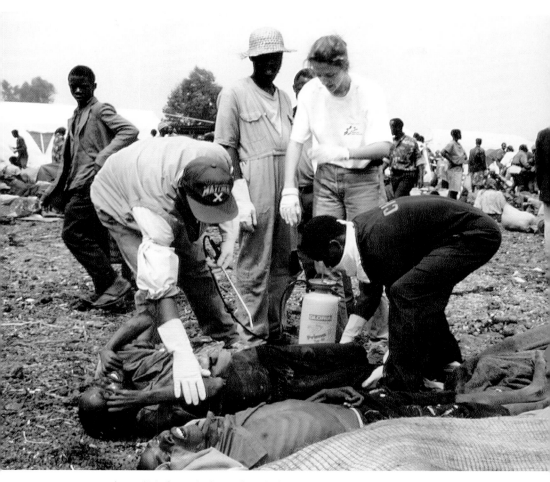

MSF workers disinfect victims of a cholera epidemic in Munigi, Zaire, in July 1994. The disease killed tens of thousands in the refugee camps that sprung up in the aftermath of the Rwandan genocide.

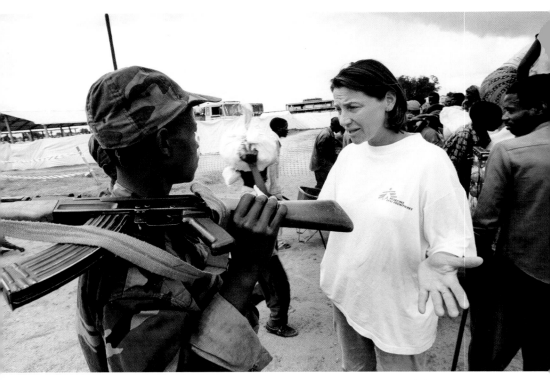

An expat pleads with an armed soldier in Kuito during Angola's civil war in September 1999. One of MSF's greatest challenges in conflict zones is negotiating access to victims on both sides.

2 | Biafra and the Bumblebee

Médecins Sans Frontières was born in a Paris boardroom in 1971, that much is certain. But the events leading up to its creation, and those surrounding its schism in 1979, have become mythical. As one French MSFer puts it mischievously, "Everybody reinvents the story in his own manner – maybe even me, too."

Everyone agrees on at least one fact of MSF's genesis: in the beginning, there was Biafra. In May 1967, a region of eastern Nigeria declared itself the independent state of Biafra, igniting a civil war. The Biafran forces had some initial success, but by early the following year, Nigerian troops had cut off supply lines to the rebel state. Soon photographs of starving children put an African famine on the international stage for the first time. Biafra waited for the world to react, but the world was preoccupied. In 1968, the United States had half a million troops in Vietnam, and the war was increasingly unpopular at home. Soviet tanks rolled into Czechoslovakia in August. And in

Paris, the dust was still settling after civil uprisings and general strikes in May. These events had the usual French trappings – barricades in the street, students singing "La Marseillaise" – but to Bernard Kouchner, it was no revolution.

Born in Avignon in 1939, Kouchner was a 29-year-old gastroenterologist with fire in his belly. Handsome, fit and self-aggrandizing, he's still a larger-than-life personality. He once lamented that he had been born too late for World War II, "too late to stop the Holocaust." *The Economist* described him this way in 1999: "Impulsive, provocative, frenetically energetic, teeming with ideas, articulate, generous and courageous, Dr. Kouchner is also blunt, abrasive, impatient, disorganised, opinionated and quick-tempered. Many have found him hard to work with ... He can appear vain and media-obsessed." Thirty years before that assessment, the doctor who would become the key founder of MSF hadn't yet developed that reputation. He was a Communist activist in Paris who came to see the student protests of May 1968 as nothing more than armchair activism. Kouchner had a grander vision for the world, and when he learned that the French Red Cross was sending volunteers to Biafra that summer, he signed up immediately, one of about 50 doctors to do so.

Most world powers sided with the Nigerian government at the time, including Britain, its former colonial power, and the Soviet Union. The United States and Egypt also weighed in on the same side, creating an unlikely four-way alliance. Only France was sympathetic to the Biafran rebels, reportedly even shipping arms to them. Kouchner's sympathies were similar, but because the Red Cross observes strict neutrality wherever it works, volunteers like Kouchner signed agreements that promised discretion. To get to the victims, he was willing to wear this muzzle, but he did so *à contrecoeur* – reluctantly.

By September, Kouchner was on his way to Biafra, flying at night to avoid being shot down. He and his colleagues then made their way by car to the village of Awo Omamma, where they found the hospital – a few decrepit buildings overflowing with hundreds of wounded men, women and children. The Red Cross doctors would also work in a feeding center a mile away, where they treated about a thousand terribly malnourished children.

The sights appalled Kouchner, who 35 years later could still recall the hungry children "like dry plants finally watered." But the French doctors soon realized that these Biafran civilians were not simply caught in the crossfire. They were being deliberately starved by the Nigerian forces, who had created a food blockade ensuring that "they would all perish, so light, so frail, in our hands." The doctors believed they were witnessing a genocide.

The Nigerian army had already shown its contempt for medical humanitarian aid. A group of Yugoslavian doctors with the Red Cross was murdered, and there were horror stories of attacks on clearly marked health centers. "They killed everyone," one Biafran told the Frenchmen, "even the doctors, nurses and hospital staff."

Kouchner eventually returned to Europe and violated the agreement he had signed with the Red Cross. With like-minded colleagues in Paris, he organized marches and media events to raise awareness of Biafra. He lobbied the international community to condemn the Nigerian government and argued that, by refusing to budge from its neutrality, the Red Cross permitted the genocide to continue. "To give medical care and keep quiet, to give medical care and let children die, for me it was clearly complicity," he told students at the

Harvard School of Public Health in 2003. "Neutrality led to complicity. The duty to interfere was born."

The idea of humanitarian intervention in the affairs of other countries has a longer tradition in France than anywhere else. In its simplest form, the concept holds that a country has the right to intervene, by force if necessary, in the affairs of another in order to prevent gross violations of human rights. Not until the mid-1980s did Bernard Kouchner – by that time long gone from MSF – try to see this "duty to interfere" enshrined in international law, but in Western Europe the idea goes back at least as far as the 17th century. British, Dutch, Belgian and German philosophers have all chimed in, but in France the idea has a particular resonance, since the French tend to think of their country as the birthplace of human rights.

The problem with humanitarian intervention, critics point out, is that, while it sounds noble, its motivation is often cynical. Colonial powers have long tried to legally justify their actions, dressing up their ambitions in moral clothing. Humanitarian intervention is also vague, both legally and morally, and full of contradictions. Countries invoke the right when it serves their foreign interests and ignore it when it doesn't. One professor of international law calls it "a joke and a fraud that has been repeatedly manipulated and abused by a small number of very powerful countries" for reasons that have nothing to do with humanitarianism. Nevertheless, by the early 20th century, it was a recognized part of French law. And so, while Biafra sparked debates about humanitarian

BIAFRA AND THE BUMBLEBEE | 45

intervention among English-speaking scholars, in France it was a *fait accompli*. This difference goes some way in explaining why MSF arose in France and not, say, in England, where the bias was toward longer-term development rather than emergency intervention.

The intellectual climate of Paris in the late 1960s also had a profound effect on the founders of MSF. Beginning in the 1950s, the former colonies of France and other European powers asserted their independence. Activists like Bernard Kouchner were inclined to support these emerging nations, despite their disillusionment with May 1968. A poster on Paris streets at the time featured a figure in riot gear beneath the words *Frontières* = *Repression*, a slogan that would soon be echoed in the name of MSF. Kouchner's generation dreamed of a new world order and hoped that humanitarianism would succeed where the left had failed.

Even the French medical system made the country ripe for an organization like MSF. Emergency medical services – the telephone-dispatched ambulances and paramedics we take for granted today – barely existed before this time. In the 1960s, France created Service d'Aide Médicale Urgente (SAMU) and trained physicians in this new field of emergency medicine. Again, this service wasn't unique – it was developing in the United States and Britain around the same time. But the French were among its pioneers, and several original and early members of Médecins Sans Frontières were doctors who had worked with SAMU.

Of course, MSF's founders brought their own personal motivations, too. As a Jewish doctor, the memory of the Holocaust – and the Red Cross's silence in the face of it – must have been an enormous influence on Kouchner. In addition, he was, and still is, well connected in French government and intellectual circles. He not only read Jean-Paul Sartre, for example, but knew him personally, and these associations lent some authority to his calls for action.

By 1970, with the war in Nigeria over, "the Biafrans," as the French doctors became known, set up an informal organization that met at Kouchner's home in Gentilly. It was clumsily named Group d'Intervention Médico-Chirurgical d'Urgence (GIMCU), and it argued – in direct opposition to the Red Cross – that the rights of victims in a conflict were more important than respecting sovereignty.

Later that year, another group of visionaries emerged in Paris, led by Raymond Borel, editor of the medical journal *Tonus*. In 1970, the journal called for French doctors to help victims of natural disasters, first in Iran, then in Yugoslavia and East Pakistan. In these cases, *Tonus* argued, international medical aid was too slow in arriving because of bureaucracy and political squabbling. Borel took up the baton and started a project called Sécours Médical Français (SMF). He put out a call for doctors.

It wasn't long before the two groups decided to join forces. After other names had been tried and found wanting, Borel came up with Médecins Sans Frontières. On December 20, 1971, amid the cigarette smoke of the *Tonus* offices, an unlikely alliance was born, one that an MSFer jokingly calls "the bastard child of a doctor and a journalist."

The two camps agreed on many things, but right away a rift opened. Kouchner and most of the Biafrans demanded that the new organization be allowed to speak out against governments if they saw the need – after all, wasn't that the reason they had broken their agreement with the Red Cross? Borel was equally adamant that they remain neutral, since no government was

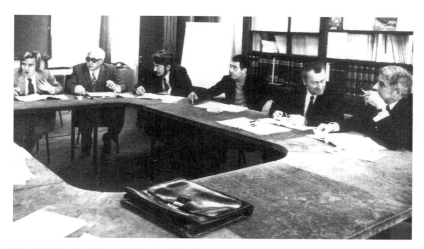

In the Paris office of the medical journal Tonus, *the founders of Médecins Sans Frontières sign the first charter on December 20, 1971. From the very beginning, the organization was divided about how and when it should speak out against the atrocities it witnessed.*

likely to risk embarrassment by opening its borders to an organization of loose cannons. As the men drew up the original MSF charter, Kouchner was forced to rein himself in – to put the *charte* before the horse. The charter's fourth article, like Kouchner's Red Cross contract three years earlier, made it clear that neutrality had won out:

> Ils respectent le secret professionnel et s'abstiennent de porter un jugement ou d'exprimer publiquement une opinion – favorable ou hostile – à l'égard des évènements, des forces et des dirigeants qui ont accepté leur concours.

> They maintain professional discretion and refrain from making judgments or expressing public opinions

– favorable or hostile – with regard to the events, forces and leaders who accepted their aid.

There were 13 men at the table that night – an omen, perhaps, of the discord that would follow.

Médecins Sans Frontières had a decidedly low profile in its first 12 months. It claimed 140 volunteers, but all were busy with regular jobs, and there were few francs in the coffers. And although MSF eventually became known for its independence and its speed in emergencies, both characteristics were still conspicuously absent. The fledgling MSF was a sort of medical human resources agency, sending doctors into the field with other aid agencies – ironically, some even worked with the Red Cross. As for being first on the scene, a key goal of Raymond Borel's, the test came days after MSF's first anniversary, when an earthquake destroyed much of Managua, Nicaragua, killing as many as 10,000 people. The organization hustled together three medical teams, including Kouchner, and sent them off with 10 tons of medical supplies. They arrived three days after the relief effort had been set up. Less than two years later, when Hurricane Fifi struck Honduras, they again failed to get there first.

More important to the future, though, was the mission that reopened the division that had begun at MSF's first meeting. In 1974, a Kurdish envoy approached Bernard Kouchner and asked MSF to support the Kurds in their rebellion in northern Iraq. Kouchner agreed, inciting the ire of Borel and his allies. Whatever personal sympathy they might have for the Kurds, the journalists argued, the dispute was within Iraqi borders, and MSF could not take sides. They pointed to the fourth article in the charter, the one that still made Kouchner seethe. After a lengthy argument, a defiant Kouchner went ahead and sent a team to Iraq, insisting his aim was purely to bring medical relief.

The provocations continued at MSF's annual assembly in February 1975, where the Biafrans and the *Tonus* members sparred openly. When the votes were counted, one of Borel's close allies lost his seat on the board, while Kouchner and a colleague took the top two posts. Now the Biafrans controlled the organization.

In its fifth year, MSF was still operating on a shoestring because its founders were reluctant to ask the public for money – fundraising methods like direct mail were unheard of in France. Still, with Kouchner at the helm, MSF saw its first successes. In 1976, it sent a rotating team of 56 volunteers to support a Beirut hospital – its first major war mission. That same year, an ad agency created a free campaign for MSF, with black-and-white print ads featuring a wide-eyed child and the words *Dans leur salle d'attente 2 milliards d'hommes* (There are two billion people in their waiting room). MSF's reputation began to grow in France and even overseas – *Time* called it "an extraordinary organization" in a report about its work in Beirut. It was even turning down young doctors who scrambled to volunteer.

But if the Biafrans felt comfortably in charge of MSF, they wouldn't for long. One of the doctors they turned away in those days was a brilliant, bespectacled 26-year-old named Rony Brauman. As the story goes, one of the veterans smiled condescendingly and said, "You know, *mon petit ami*, in Beirut

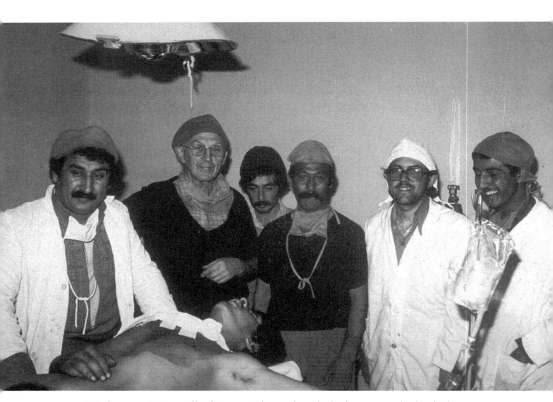

A Lebanese MSF medical team takes a break during a surgical mission in the late 1970s. While its successes were modest in the early years, MSF won international acclaim in 1976 when Time *magazine called it "an extraordinary organization" for its efforts in Lebanon.*

we're dodging bullets." In the years to come, Brauman would make the old boys dodge a few bullets of his own.

The world changed in the late 1970s, and MSF changed with it. As people fled wars in Southeast Asia, Africa, and Central and South America, the number of refugees doubled between

1976 and 1979 to almost 6 million people. Before this period, MSF carried out most of its missions in conflict zones or natural disasters, but now a new breed of emergency physician was finding a role – the refugee camp doctor.

Claude Malhuret was among the first MSF doctors to work in Thailand with refugees fleeing the killing fields of Cambodia. Ten years younger than Kouchner but already balding, with a bushy mustache that hid his upper lip, the 26-year-old quickly earned respect for his courage and hard work. Malhuret wasted no time in articulating a new vision for MSF, one that included longer-term missions and better organization. His team in Thailand often had enough medical supplies, but they were ripping open cardboard boxes in a chaotic warehouse to find what they needed. They also lacked people who could arrange food, shelter and cars and tend to administrative tasks, so the doctors could concentrate on their patients.

In April 1977, Kouchner himself praised Malhuret at MSF's annual assembly, where the newcomer was elected head of the Paris office. Within months, though, the two began to lock horns. Soon the battle lines were clearly drawn between *le clan Biafrais* and *le bande de Cochin*, those of Malhuret's generation, who took their nickname from the Paris university they attended. By 1978, the debates grew fierce, with the latter group insisting that if MSF was ever going to become more than a rabble of amateurs – what the French call *bricolage* – it would have to improve its logistics and learn to raise funds. The founders, meanwhile, saw their vision being hijacked by a bunch of upstarts who wanted to turn the movement into an overly technical medical delivery service. The dispute about whether volunteers should be able to speak publicly about their missions continued as well. The Biafrans had managed to get the controversial article removed from the charter in 1977, but Malhuret's group, like Borel's, was wary of denouncing governments in areas where MSF worked.

Looking back, it sounds like a tidy division, but nothing in MSF is ever simple. "It's easier to put it that way thirty years later," says Rony Brauman, who sided with Malhuret early on, was president of MSF's French office from 1982 to 1994, and is still the movement's philosopher-king. "We knew what we *didn't* want: We didn't want to continue with this very amateur medicine – just being there with some drugs in a plastic bag and a few surgical tools. What we brought was not more intelligence or more open-mindedness. It's just that we were not prisoners of the dreams of the founders."

Board meetings soon became confrontations that could last until three in the morning. At opposite ends of the table, Kouchner gestured dramatically while Malhuret hunched over his papers and countered every argument with his own. Before one of these legendary Gallic duels, Kouchner held the boardroom door for Malhuret and said, "Welcome to the arena." Patrick Aeberhard, one of the Biafrans who remains a friend and supporter of Kouchner today, remembers that the power balance shifted quickly to the Cochin group. "They took over the organization in a weekend. They arrived with a very pushy, political way in this organization, which was at the time very informal."

The disagreements simmered until the final weeks of 1978, when TV audiences around the world watched a tragedy unfold in the China Sea. Since the fall of Saigon in 1975, hundreds of thousands of boat people had fled Vietnam on whatever suspect vessels they could find. In November, unwilling to deal with more refugees, Malaysia turned away the *Hai Kong*, a ship carrying some 2,500 Vietnamese. Sanitary conditions on

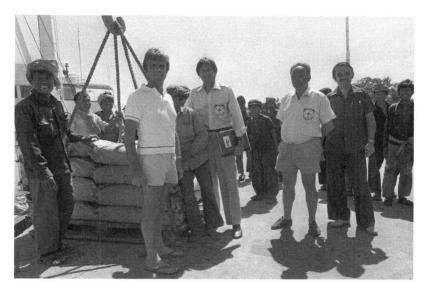

After cutting ties with MSF in 1979, Bernard Kouchner stayed in the spotlight as founder of the aid group Médecins du Monde, as a prominent politician in France, and as head of the UN mission in Kosovo. He continues to visit the world's high-profile crises – and never forgets to bring a camera crew.

the ship – packed so tightly there was no room to lie down – were unspeakable. Cameras caught an image of the desperate passengers holding a banner over the rails with the words *Please rescue us.*

The banner spurred Bernard Kouchner into action. Within days he formed a committee called "A Boat for Vietnam" and chartered a ship, *L'Île de Lumière,* with the idea of transporting the fleeing Vietnamese safely to a new country. But when the committee asked MSF to look after medical services on the ship, the organization split along predictable lines. Kouchner's opponents pointed out the obvious flaws in the mission. One ship would be hopelessly inadequate – in November alone, the number of people fleeing Vietnam peaked at 21,500. Worse, they argued, the mission might encourage more refugees to risk the open seas and the pirates that had already claimed the lives of thousands.

The affair was personal, too, of course, and it was really only a catalyst. Malhuret and Borel had long grown tired of Kouchner's histrionics and love of the limelight. At a meeting to discuss the mission on November 28, 1978, the feud came to a head. Kouchner, Aeberhard and their supporters knew they were outnumbered and, after a heated exchange, they stormed out of the room.

L'Île de Lumière sailed as planned, but not under the flag of MSF. Kouchner and his team used the vessel as a hospital ship, tending to some 40,000 refugees. Whatever MSF thought of the mission, it was given the Prix Louise Weiss, an annual award in France that recognizes contributions to peace and human relations. The Cochin clan, meanwhile, worked hard to drum up support for Malhuret, criticizing Kouchner at every turn. MSF's annual assembly on May 5, 1979, was clearly going to be the final showdown. At the Paris Hilton that day, Malhuret praised the new direction MSF had taken, including longer-term missions in refugee camps. Kouchner countered by saying that by opposing *L'Île de Lumière*, a mission that MSF was born to do, the organization had lost sight of its ideals. "The MSF label does not belong to those who simply wear the badge but to a spirit and a moral, to an honor." Clearly their visions of MSF were incompatible and it went to a vote. Of the 120 ballots cast, 90 came back in favor of Malhuret. The coup was complete.

Kouchner and his allies left the assembly in disgust, never to return. Patrick Aeberhard, who followed Kouchner out the door, remembers the feeling as he turned his back. "We were betrayed."

Exactly what went on behind closed doors in those heady days of 1979 is preserved only in the selective memories of the people who were there. History, as they say, is written by the victors, and the official MSF version today reads like the triumph of pragmatic realists over a group of passionate but naïve and grandstanding visionaries.

After Bernard Kouchner's departure, the new leaders – especially Claude Malhuret and Rony Brauman – worked quickly to make MSF more professional, knowing it could not rely on sporadic donations. Within a year, they almost tripled the organization's budget, and in 1982 they introduced direct-mail fundraising and began paying a small stipend to doctors who did long-term missions. But this was no group of technocrats, and MSF's activities after the schism were, ironically, even bolder than those of the Kouchner years. They pushed the limits of neutrality – and did some grandstanding of their own.

After the Soviets invaded Afghanistan in December 1979, MSF was the first agency on the scene, entering the country illegally and exposing its volunteers to grave danger. It made no pretense of neutrality: medical aid went to the mujahideen, the Afghan resistance fighters. "There was never any question as to whether MSF should offer its services in Kabul in order to be able to sit on the fence," Brauman wrote later. "Like our forerunners in Biafra, we had implicitly picked our side. We all saw it as our duty to expose the scale of this war to the world." The new leadership was sounding like the founders they had just expelled. And while Kouchner's critics had lamented his penchant for media stunts, MSF's first public denunciation of a government was a march led by celebrities, including singer Joan Baez and actress Liv Ullmann. Staged in February 1980, the march was an unsuccessful attempt to bring medical aid across the Thailand–Cambodia border to aid victims of the brutal Khmer Rouge. Brauman himself was one of the marchers, and he acknowledged that MSF "fully realised that they were kissing goodbye any prospect of being able to operate in the country after their act of provocation."

It's going too far to argue that the generation of Malhuret and Brauman ousted MSF's founders and then promptly reverted to Kouchner's old ideas. Humanitarian aid has always been reactive, responding to the political climate in the world at large. To this day, many of MSF's principles are fluid concepts that, necessarily, evolve according to what's happening around them. Brauman argues that it was MSF's experience in the refugee camps of that period – 90 percent of the camp populations were fleeing Communist rule – that forced it to speak out against totalitarian regimes. At the same time, MSF began to overcome many of the technical inadequacies it had experienced as a young organization, something the old guard seemed unable to do. But in the coming years, MSF emerged on the world stage not because of its logistical ability but because it was a brash and fearless group that went where others would not go.

Médecins Sans Frontières finally expanded out of France in 1980, with the addition of a small office in Brussels, followed by another in Geneva in 1981. Even this modest expansion didn't come without growing pains. One of those to go on mission with the young Belgian section was Jacques de Milliano, a

Dutch doctor who traveled to Chad in 1983, during the war between Muslim northerners and Christians from the south. In February, he was part of a convoy when one of the trucks ahead of him hit a mine, seriously wounding three people, all southerners. One had both lower legs blown off, and de Milliano used a stick and a piece of string to stop the bleeding the best he could, burying the severed limbs in the sand. When de Milliano was still a half-hour from stabilizing his patients, a Muslim commander named Mussa told him that his time was up and the convoy had to move on. De Milliano recalled the discussion in his journal: "'To you northerners, the life of a southerner has no value whatsoever,' I replied, 'but we are doctors and we treat everyone – or no one. That includes the wounded people from your tribe in the back of the lorries. The choice is up to you.' Mussa turned round and ordered the drivers to wait."

After returning to Holland, de Milliano and several other doctors met in the basement of an Amsterdam canal house every Thursday evening and soon hatched a plan to start an MSF section in their own country. The Belgians were supportive, but, de Milliano remembers, "the French didn't like the idea. All those new clubs bearing the same name. How could they check whether they operated according to the same principles?"

Undaunted, the group established MSF-Holland on September 7, 1984. A few weeks later, the French agreed to recognize it, and the newly minted section opened an office in Amsterdam with one full-time employee.

The following year, after a billion people watched Bob Geldof's televised Live Aid concerts for famine relief, MSF watched Ethiopia's Communist dictator, Colonel Mengistu, abuse that aid. With the vehicles, cash and food he received from international donors, Mengistu moved people from the drought-ravaged north to the more fertile south. On the surface, the plan seemed logical, but soon it became clear that Mengistu was using the promise of food to uproot people against their will, often with the consent of aid organizations – some were not allowed to distribute food to hungry children unless their parents agreed to the resettlement plan. But because the organizations wanted to remain in Ethiopia and help where they could, they kept silent – including MSF-Belgium. The French section, however, publicly denounced the Mengistu regime and was promptly expelled from the country in December 1985. The gesture wasn't futile – shortly afterward, the European Community and the United States insisted that the deportations had to stop if Ethiopia was to receive more international relief.

Back in Europe, MSF was having civil strife of its own. In 1984, Brauman, Malhuret and others launched Liberté Sans Frontières, a sort of political arm of MSF. The young Belgian section – at the time regarded by the French as merely *une filiale*, a subsidiary – objected noisily to this new foundation, which it saw as a threat to MSF's neutrality. The following year, relations strained further after the sections disagreed over how to respond in Ethiopia, and the Paris office launched a lawsuit to try to prevent the Belgians from using the MSF name. It failed, LSF dissolved shortly afterward, and today Brauman calls the suit an "enormous error."

These days, some commentators still describe MSF as the cowboys of emergency aid, a label the organization discourages. During the 1980s, however, it was more appropriate. Some of the stories from that era beggar belief, including the one related by Peter Dalglish in *The Courage of Children*. Dalglish, the founder of Street Kids International, would become one of the key people in establishing the Canadian section of MSF. In March 1987, he was working for UNICEF in Wau, in the predominantly Dinka region of South Sudan. Dalglish had become friends with Jacques de Milliano and suggested that MSF-Holland provide medical support to the Wau hospital, after UNICEF deemed the assignment too dangerous. MSF obliged and sent two Dutch doctors, whom Dalglish calls Harry and Marijke.

When the team arrived to assess the mission, Wau was so volatile and isolated that Dalglish said they should forget the whole thing, but Harry and Marijke insisted on staying. One of the town's policemen offered to show them how to fire a gun, then stood back in amazement as Harry pumped five bullets into the bull's-eye – he had neglected to tell the MSF recruiters that he was a former commando with the Dutch army. In any case, the doctors figured that if it became necessary, they could always evacuate with the one pilot brazen enough to fly supplies into the town.

Two weeks later, that pilot was shot down on his way to Wau. Now no one could get in, and Harry and Marijke had no way out – and another two weeks passed before anyone heard from them. Finally, a messenger rode 125 miles on his bike to deliver a note explaining that the doctors' radio had been stolen. He warned that an out-of-control military commander named Abu Gurun was mercilessly hunting Dinka civilians around Wau.

It was nine months before a UNICEF plane finally got Harry and Marijke out, and by this time Harry was clearly traumatized. Abu Gurun and his troops had tortured, mutilated and executed the Dinka with unimaginable cruelty. They cut off genitals, forced children to murder their own parents, machine-gunned people by the hundreds, herded them into a storeroom and gassed them with carbon monoxide. One day Harry came across the bodies of eight children impaled on spears. Another night, he was invited to the commander's home for dinner and, as he ate a dish of meat and gravy, he recognized a human joint among the bones. It was the last straw for Harry:

> He would reciprocate Abu Gurun's hospitality by inviting him to dinner at the doctors' residence. The meal would require some careful preparation: the MSF doctor planned to inject ... live cholera culture into the food just minutes before it was served. Harry had the pharmaceuticals necessary to treat cholera and would take a dose to protect himself against the effects of the disease. He expected that Abu Gurun, after having consumed the pasta dinner, would be writhing in pain before breakfast the next day. His death would be suitably miserable.

The plane arrived before he could carry out his plan.

Harry and Marijke's experience in South Sudan was extreme and not at all typical of MSF's activities at that time or any other. MSF discourages former military personnel from volunteering and has never allowed its people to carry a weapon, to say nothing of Harry's vigilante cookery. But it's a snapshot from an era when the organization really did go into situations that every other agency avoided. MSF is still active today in South Sudan, but by current standards Wau would have been deemed too risky for a pair of expat doctors without their own vehicles, nothing more than a VHF radio for communication, and the only support team more than 600 miles away in Khartoum.

"Over the years," Dalglish could still write in 1998, "employees of MSF have become inured to the sight of UN employees and their families standing in long lines in airports around the world with their suitcases at their sides, at the very moment MSF personnel are arriving to begin their emergency work." Today, the organization still works in isolated areas where no one else is delivering medical aid and goes to its share of dangerous places. But if the situation is so precarious that other aid agencies are pulling out, MSF will usually join them – at least temporarily, until the authorities can guarantee their safety. This caution isn't institutional cowardice – it's simply the reality of delivering aid in places where a cavalier attitude will get you killed.

By the late 1980s, MSF's reputation had spread throughout Europe. Spain and Luxembourg had opened offices in 1986, bringing the number of national sections to six, and variations of the organization's logo now bore the names Artsen Zonder Grenzen and Medicos Sin Fronteras. In 1989, a group of pollsters asked the French public to name their dream job, and the most popular answer – 32 percent – was to work for MSF.

The organization still had a low profile in English-speaking countries, however, and that would remain so until the new decade. Here again, MSF seemed less than eager to grow outside Europe. In April 1989, Canadian doctor Richard Heinzl flew to Paris to meet with Francis Charhon, one of the leaders of MSF-France. "I wanted to talk to the French about trying to

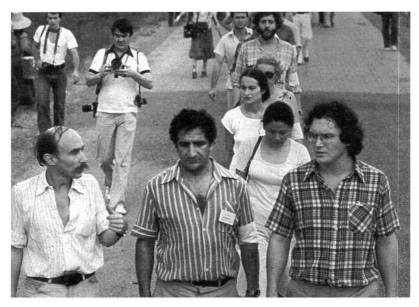

MSF's new generation was headed by doctors Claude Malhuret, Xavier Emmanuelli and Rony Brauman, shown here leading the March for the Survival of Cambodia in February 1980. It was the group's first témoignage, or advocacy campaign.

get the movement over here," Heinzl remembers. "When I arrived, Charhon was standing there with his white hair, smoking this Cuban cigar, and he didn't even remember inviting me, and he was shocked that I was there. I said, 'We've got to do it, Canada's right for this, we're French and English, we believe in it.' And he basically just gave me a flat no. Then, puffing on his big cigar, he winked and said, 'But if you have the will ...' That's all I needed to hear."

The United States beat Heinzl to the punch, though, opening its New York office in 1990, followed by Canada in 1991, with both new sections generally being referred to, at least by the public, as Doctors Without Borders. (It's interesting to note that virtually everyone in the organization now shuns the English name.) By 1995, MSF had sections in Australia, the United Kingdom, Germany, Austria, Italy, Denmark, Sweden, Norway, Japan, Hong Kong and Greece. Today, the offices in France, Belgium, Holland, Switzerland and Spain are the operational sections – every MSF field mission is administered by at least one of these privileged five. Each of the other 13 offices, called partner sections, is paired with one of the operational countries – the US section with France, the Canadians with Holland, the Scandinavians with Belgium, and so on. The main role of the partner sections is fundraising and recruiting volunteers for their operational parent, as well as raising public awareness in their home countries. The US section – MSF's cash cow, having raised about $55 million from American citizens in 2003 – began running joint operations with France in 2004. Otherwise, MSF is doing its best to keep its partner sections content without giving them operational responsibilities, lest it become a beast with 18 heads.

MSF's world headquarters is in Geneva, and its coordinating body is called the International Council – it comprises the heads of each of the sections, plus an international president. Exactly how much power this council wields depends on whom you talk to, but it certainly isn't intended to issue decrees to the operational sections, all of which have a large degree of autonomy. MSF considers itself not a formal top-down organization, but a movement of like-minded members.

Each of the big five headquarters has its distinct culture, style and personality, and these differences play out in colorful ways. "You have to see a fight between sections to understand what it is to be MSF," says a veteran doctor who has worked with three of them. There is the danger of stereotypes, but what you hear over and over from experienced MSFers is often the same – the French are passionate but arrogant and disorganized (the UN's Stephen Lewis once described them as "amiably deranged"), the Dutch are the technical wizards, the Belgians are somewhere in between. A nurse sums it up this way: "If you hang out with the Dutch, you know you're going to have endless meetings. If you hang out with the French, you know you're going to get good cheese and good wine."

The MSF brass tends to downplay these differences or dismiss them as outdated relics. It's true that in the last five or six years, after MSF stopped adding new national sections and allowed the existing ones to mature, it has become more coherent, even as it becomes more cosmopolitan. And as more volunteers come from non-European countries, the sections are less likely to mirror their national cultures. MSFers in the field are still overwhelmingly European, however. Of the 3,000 or so who go abroad in a typical year, roughly 800 are citizens of France. Belgium (a country of only 10 million) sends about 400; Holland and Spain, 200 each; and the United Kingdom about 150. Australia contributes about 110, while Canada had almost 140 in the field at the end of 2003. The United States, despite a population that's double that of MSF's five operational countries combined, and ten times that of Canada, sent 135 expats on mission in 2003. (One reason for these disproportionate numbers is that francophone Canadians – almost half the volunteers are from the province of Quebec – slip easily into MSF's culture. Another is that American volunteers may be more difficult to place in parts of the world where the US military is active.) A smaller number of Latin Americans, Africans and Asians round out the expat lineup.

Many MSFers are happy to bid goodbye to the national chauvinism. "I didn't grow up in France, or Belgium, or Holland," says an American logistician who had little patience for the sectional squabbling he saw during his missions. "For me, it was just dismay seeing all this wasted energy: 'The French are this, the Dutch are that, the Belgians are this.' Who gives a shit?" What the organization has retained is a deeply entrenched culture of debate, of reexamining everything it does. "We still fight like hell," says Austen Davis, executive director of MSF-Holland, "but we fight over much smaller things now."

MSF's structure appears inefficient – in Angola and Afghanistan, where all five operational sections have worked simultaneously, it might have five heads of mission, in five offices, with 10 cars. But each will have its own responsibilities, and the sections avoid overlap. Besides, Davis says, the model allows MSF to be creative. "One of the chief challenges to humanitarian action is getting access to victims. It's a very entrepreneurial business, and putting all your eggs in one basket and having a monolithic structure isn't as conducive as floating around a crisis with lots of little groups, lots of little teams, lots of contacts, trying different things." In some cases, one section may fall out of favor with authorities, while another is welcomed to continue the work. The sections have also evolved their own specialties – Holland tends to focus on conflict zones, for example, while Belgium has the most experience with AIDS programs.

"Aerodynamically, the bumblebee shouldn't be able to fly," says an often-quoted bit of wisdom, "but the bumblebee doesn't know it, so it goes on flying anyway." It turns out that's an entomological urban legend, but it endures because we like the paradox of something that shouldn't work, but does. MSF is just this kind of bumblebee: renowned for its ability to act quickly, despite having no clear central authority. Tine Dusauchoit, general director of the Belgian section, admits: "It doesn't make sense unless you know MSF, and you *see* that it functions."

Part of the reason the bumblebee can stay airborne is that there's money holding it up. Yet when you consider the scope of its activities around the world, MSF's budget isn't enormous – about $400 million – and most comes from private donations. (By way of comparison, World Vision's US branch alone spent over $1 billion in 2002.) Overall, MSF draws only about 20 percent of its funds from the United Nations High Commissioner for Refugees (UNHCR), the European Commission's Humanitarian Aid Office (ECHO) and governments, the pork barrels of most aid agencies. Through a combination of shrewd fundraising, frugality and a reliance on low-paid staff or unpaid volunteers, MSF thrives largely on the checks that arrive each month from private citizens.

Other aid agencies – particularly those that rely on child sponsorship programs, such as Save the Children, World Vision and Plan International – may give the impression that they rely heavily on donations from the public, but in reality they are far more dependent on government agencies. MSF was, too, until it made a movement-wide goal to get away from it. The organization feels that dependence on UN and government donors is a trap – it forces aid agencies to become institutionalized, too bureaucratic and too unwilling to bite the hands that feed them. Other agencies, not surprisingly, are not impressed with the implications of that argument.

"There's definitely a sense among some organizations that MSF is a pain in the ass – and MSF *is* a pain in the ass, very often," says Kenny Gluck, operations director for MSF-Holland, who gained some perspective when he worked with other non-governmental organizations, including the International Rescue Committee. "There is some jealously in it. I was mostly jealous, when I was at IRC, of MSF's ability to move first and think about money later. We can slam the donors. They can't, because they're getting too much money from them. If the governmental donors want to yank our funding, fine, we have a base of support in the public, which other organizations don't have, or they don't value. CARE has it, but instead of guarding their independence, they use their private base to get more government funding to become bigger. We've chosen not to do that. They can be jealous, but it was a strategic choice by them as an organization to be very big, and it was a strategic choice by us to stay small but be independent."

In the field, aid organizations complain that MSF can seem aloof. One UNICEF employee remembers offering to help a nervous-looking young MSFer in some African airport and hearing her respond, "No thanks, I'm not supposed to associate with other aid agencies." More significantly, they've been accused of being unwilling to coordinate with other agencies – a charge MSF admits to unabashedly, though it stresses it's never on technical grounds, and it's not about guarding its turf. MSF wants to be in the loop, but not in the noose. "To the extent that the military are there, or UNHCR is there, or ECHO is there doing a great job, we'll work alongside them. But we will not subsume ourselves to their project," Austen Davis says. "They do things that we can't do, and they do things that we want to happen. But we want to retain the positive critical analysis to be able to scream and shout when they fuck up."

That's the thing about bumblebees – sometimes they sting.

3 | We Don't Need Another Hero

People who choose to live or work outside their home society – whether intrepid explorers, cloistered monks or humanitarian aid workers – have always exerted a strong pull on the cultures they've left behind. That may be why MSF volunteers are commonly asked, "Why do you do this kind of work?"

The query annoys most of them, not only because of its tiresome frequency but because motivations are difficult to distill into a concise answer. They also worry they might disappoint the questioner, who has usually assumed that aid work is a hair shirt, an act of self-sacrifice. As one doctor puts it: "People hear about MSF and say, 'You're going to be nominated for sainthood,' and it's not at all like that. I consider myself a person after his own self-interests. It's rewarding to bring medical care to these people, but I'm doing it because it makes me feel good, and I like it. I'm not doing it for them – I mean, I am, but I go there because it feels right for me, not because I think I'm helping the world."

That's not to downplay the genuine altruism that motivates all MSF volunteers on some level. It's just that the degree to which it plays a part varies dramatically, even in the same person over time. The drive to do that first mission is rarely the same as the one that prompts a fifth or sixth visit to the field.

Many MSFers can recall the moment when the idea of humanitarian work crystallized in their mind. For family physician Andrew Schechtman, who has done missions in Guatemala and Liberia, it came in a university library, where he was procrastinating instead of studying for an undergraduate test. "I picked up an old book on the table next to me and started looking through it, and it turned out to be one of Albert Schweitzer's books about the jungle hospital in Lambaréné, in Gabon. It just hit home – the type of work he was doing, where he was the only doctor in that hospital, taking care of people who had no other access to care. That clinched my idea to go into medicine, and it also planted the seed of wanting to do overseas work further down the road."

Growing up during the Cultural Revolution in China, pediatric surgeon Wei Cheng was inspired by a different medical icon. Cheng's childhood hero was Norman Bethune, the Canadian surgeon who assisted the Chinese during the Japanese invasion in 1938. In November the following year, Bethune, operating without gloves, pricked his finger and contracted septicemia. Without antibiotics, he died from the infection and was given a hero's burial, with Mao Tse-tung delivering the eulogy. "People of my generation still respect him very much," says Cheng, who in 2000 became the first Hong Kong surgeon to volunteer with MSF.

Vincent Echave, a Cuban-born surgeon in his mid-60s, also grew up during a Communist revolution, where he first came face to face with suffering in his own country. "Then, traveling around the world, I realized that a doctor's mission is not only to cure people and make money here but to give something of his time and knowledge to poor people. It's a deep conviction of mine that it is essential for any human being, but especially a doctor, to give part of his time to humanitarian work."

Even if most physicians share Echave's sentiments, MSF's keenest challenge is finding enough doctors. The organization requires one or two years (depending on the section) of clinical experience, so freshly minted MDs aren't eligible, let alone the medical students who often inquire and are surprised to find that MSF doesn't take all comers. For many young doctors carrying enormous debts from their student loans – especially in the United States, less so in Europe – humanitarian aid work can seem like a luxury they can't afford. For more experienced doctors with thriving practices, the inability to find locums during their absence can be just as prohibitive. First missions usually last six to nine months, since the learning curve is steepest for newcomers. Those who make subsequent trips to the field may stay for shorter periods.

The average age of MSF expats is 37 years, but that's misleading. If you visit a field project, you'll find that most non-medical people, in particular, are considerably younger, so the overall mean is probably distorted by older doctors doing short missions. Humanitarian aid work mainly attracts single, childless people, so, by their late 30s, those inclined to start a family have usually found less adventurous employers or, if they stay with MSF, exchanged field missions for office jobs.

Whatever their age, doctors who volunteer with MSF don't all fit the same mold. Some manage to interrupt their practices to do emergency missions for a few weeks each year.

Others devote most of their careers to aid work, having always known they were most comfortable caring for patients largely forgotten by others. In addition to her work with MSF, family physician Leslie Shanks has treated tuberculosis in the Canadian Arctic, worked in remote Native communities, cared for federal prisoners, and now works in a clinic in the heart of Toronto's gay community. "A nightmare for me would be to work in a standard suburban practice, talking to people about their ill-fitting orthotics and treating sore throats," says Shanks. "That, to me, is my worst nightmare. I'm extremely fortunate to be in the field that I'm in because, as a family doc, I have all kinds of opportunity to do interesting things where I actually feel like I'm contributing something – usually not a lot, but a small bit. Working in an area that is overserviced, I just couldn't do that. I have no patience for it."

For others, the push comes later, when they begin to look for new challenges after practicing in the increasingly specialized world of Western medicine. With so many experts available to their patients, general practitioners are far more likely to give a referral than to try an unfamiliar procedure, which is good for the patient but less rewarding for a doctor. For their part, specialists may be looking to add some variety to their own experience. "There's huge appeal to the scope of medicine you get to practice," Schechtman says. "I had to do things I really wasn't trained to do, but there was nobody better to do them. It was sort of a MacGyver situation, where I had to just do my best with the training and tools I had. It challenged me as a doctor to push myself to the limits, and I learned a lot because of that."

MSF tries to match its medical staff to the needs of each project, but circumstances sometimes mess up those plans. In the Liberian hospital where Schechtman worked, the local surgeon disappeared for a month and left him on his own. One of his first patients was a woman in labor whose baby had become stuck. "There was no alternative than to try and get this baby out. I did a Cesarean section, and she had a ruptured uterus that I couldn't repair, so I had to do a hysterectomy also. I was definitely in way over my head. I had done maybe fifteen Cesarean sections in residency, six years before, and maybe five hysterectomies, but always with a senior physician standing across the table and telling me where to put my scissor and how deep to cut. It was really stressful, but the only other option would have been to just watch. She ended up doing well."

One motivating factor is particularly acute among American doctors: lawsuits. "The biggest thing I found when I first went overseas was that there was this huge load lifted off my shoulders – all this malpractice threat that Western physicians, particularly in the US, have to work under," says one surgeon. "That constant threat that every time you make a decision you're looking over your shoulder for a lawyer. I was immensely relieved that was gone."

While surgeons are an exception, many first-time doctors and nurses are surprised to find that an MSF project may involve little direct treatment of patients. "The thing we're looking for among medical people is an understanding that you're not going to get involved with too much individual patient care," says an MSF recruiter. "You've got to get that out of your mind, because it's not going to be as hands-on as you think. You're a lot more effective using ten local health-care workers than trying to do it all yourself. That's a bit tough for people, because you're suddenly entering management, computers, statistics, reports, and that's not always what doctors want."

Nurses, too, find that MSF gives them far more responsibility than they would get in a typical Western setting. "I couldn't give Tylenol without a physician's order," says Kathleen Bochsler, a nurse who worked in a remote northern Canadian community before going to Kandahar, Afghanistan. "Technically, at three o'clock in the morning if my patient needed Tylenol, I had to phone a physician and wake him or her up. That's just ridiculous. We're supposed to be intelligent enough and trained enough to make life-saving decisions, yet I can't give Tylenol? It's very frustrating, especially if you've worked independently, without a physician, and you're making some important decisions on your own, to have to go back to working in an environment where your opinion is always secondary."

Nonmedical people, too, are attracted by the promise of challenge. Remembering his first mission in Somalia, an MSF administrator says he got to sit in on meetings with UN and military staff, handle about $40,000 a month in cash, and do much of the radio communications with Mogadishu and Nairobi. "It was a great job for someone in their mid-twenties. Every day was different, and there were some days that were absolutely incredible. I was doing a lot of things I never imagined I could do."

Though Médecins Sans Frontières prides itself on having remained small relative to development agencies like CARE or World Vision, it's hardly the ragtag group it was in the 1970s. Yet it has always struggled to stay close to those roots, beginning with the French reluctance to expand to Belgium and Holland in the 1980s. In his Nobel Prize acceptance speech,

James Orbinski, then MSF's international president, went so far as to say, "MSF is not a formal institution, and with any luck at all, it never will be."

In mid-October 1999, there were small but boisterous parties all over the world, as field staff toasted the announcement that MSF had been awarded the Nobel Peace Prize. There were celebrations in the European and North American offices, too, of course, but also uneasiness. "I remember the day we received the Nobel Prize I was really worrying about the effects it would have," says Jean-Hervé Bradol, president of MSF-France. "I thought there would be a danger of taking ourselves too seriously, of trying to play in the courtyard of the really big players on international issues." Bradol was worried that MSF would be thrust onto the stage and asked to speak out on issues that aren't directly related to humanitarian medical assistance. "If you have a meeting about an issue that you are not really involved in – for instance, the death penalty – you will have people saying, 'An organization like MSF, with the Nobel Prize, should have a public position on that.'"

Five years later, Bradol and most other MSFers have made peace with the prize – if nothing else, adding "Nobel Laureate" to its stationery has been a godsend for fundraising. However, Kenny Gluck of MSF-Holland recognizes that it has had a lingering effect on recruiting. "Different kinds of people join us now that we're big and famous. When you're little, scrappy and rebellious, different kinds of people come forward to be volunteers."

Even before the Nobel Prize, MSF tried to ensure that at least 30 percent of its expats were first-timers, to guard against attracting too many complacent career volunteers. Gluck admits that "everyone else in the humanitarian movement makes fun of us" for this policy, which can lead to inexperienced people being overwhelmed by too much responsibility. But even second-time volunteers admit that nothing compares to the urgency of a first mission, that baptism of fire in a hospital on the edge of a war zone. "There's a shock of transition between the shiny clean urban hospital and one where there's trauma you've never seen, where health care has abominably low standards. That shock is a driving force in the organization. It also allows a person to tell an old fart like me, 'I don't give a damn that you've seen twenty places that are worse than this. This offends me, and I want to do something about it.' That's what we try to institutionalize as a check against our own cynicism, against the thick skin we develop."

As an organization – those who share Orbinski's hope prefer the term *movement* – MSF is relatively nonhierarchical (except in the field, where a chain of command is essential) and egalitarian. All volunteers are invited to join the association – there's one in each country with an MSF section – which allows them to vote for board members or run for a position on that board. And unlike many UK and US charities that are chaired by the gentry or by captains of industry, MSF boards are composed of former field volunteers, many of them doctors. "We try to structure the organization so that everyone owns it," says Austen Davis. "So if it's not performing well, they can't just complain about the boss. It's their responsibility to speak up and say where MSF should go in the future, and to get a personal sense of ownership and commitment in the work they're doing."

Field volunteers are paid a small stipend, which varies according to the MSF section, the position, and the person's experience – first-timers may receive less than $1,000 a month, while an eight-year veteran managing all the field missions in a country might make three times that amount. The organization picks up all travel costs and health insurance, but expats pay for their own food and most other expenses in the field. Even MSF's office staff is paid modestly, and equitably, compared with private companies. At MSF's New York office, for example, the ratio of highest to lowest salary is not more than three to one, with the executive director making about $94,000. When hiring local staff in the field, however, MSF's tendency is to pay slightly more than the going rate among other NGOs.

Because even the top jobs aren't going to make you rich, MSF attracts many people who are congenitally uncomfortable amid the affluence of the West. Martin Girard has done missions in Colombia, Sierra Leone, the Democratic Republic of Congo and Sudan, and now recruits volunteers at MSF's Montreal office. "There's no way I could work in the private sector, unless I was totally broke and I needed a job that pays more," he says. "But I'm not attached to material things. I'm forty years old and I don't have a car. I don't have the money for it. My mother and father paid for the washer and dryer in my new apartment, because I didn't have the money for it.

"If I sent my CV to the UN tomorrow morning, I can assure you I would have a job, at perhaps five thousand dollars a month," continues Girard, who has a master's degree in political science, is fluent in three languages, and has traveled in more than two dozen countries. "But I know that I would be losing part of my soul in a big political organization, having to make compromises in the field that I can't accept."

Girard has little patience for people who romanticize humanitarian aid work. "I've had one or two yuppies come into my office, saying: 'I've made all my money, and I've got my big house. My life is a total wreck, and I think I would find meaning if I went on a mission with you.' I ask them, 'Would you be happier if I sent you to a genocide? Do you think you're going to come back and smile at the sun every morning? Do you think that's the recipe for happiness? The expats we sent to Rwanda in 1994 are still seeing the shrink once a week.'"

No one really knows what to expect on that first mission. Pediatric emergency doctor Joanne Liu remembers reading a book about MSF when she was 13 years old and dreaming of doing humanitarian work when she grew up. "I did my first mission when I was thirty – that's a long time to carry a dream. Of course, I was doomed to face disappointment, because my expectations were so high. I could not believe the bureaucracy of humanitarian aid work. I just could not understand it." Liu did her first mission in Mauritania, where refugees were getting set to return to neighboring Mali. She says a UN official there was trying to move the refugees during the rainy season, just to make himself look good by getting them closer to the border. "Of course, he didn't order enough plastic sheeting, and the people ended up living under the rain for another two weeks. We had increased mortality, diarrhea, upper-respiratory infections. I could not believe that because this person had an agenda, he was willing to put the health of forty thousand refugees at stake. I was really naïve, and my head of mission told me, 'Joanne, wake up. Welcome to this world, honey.' I remember writing letters to my parents and my significant other, saying I cannot believe this, and I can't believe MSF is not fighting it. I was so disappointed and I didn't think I'd ever go again. I'd been dreaming about this for seventeen years, and this is what I have to deal with?"

After four years practicing law, followed by an MBA, Patrick Lemieux had a dream of his own – to find a job where he could get some real sense that he was helping others. "I was in Barcelona at that point, so I contacted MSF-Spain, and it was very quick. I did two interviews and I was off to Kosovo. I took care of finance, logistics and administration, and while I was there, the team decided to close down the entire mission. So in six months I shut down two projects. It had nothing to do with the feel-good work I was hoping to do. I was freezing my balls off in Kosovo, spending Christmas by myself, firing people, arguing about contracts, and liquidating assets. I did enjoy the experience of being in that area, and obviously you develop relationships with the national staff. Definitely some nice moments, but it wasn't what I thought it would be."

What's surprising is not the ingenuous notions of first-time volunteers but their willingness to persevere. After her disaster in Mauritania, Liu has done more than a dozen missions with MSF, and Lemieux is approaching double digits, too. With experience, humanitarian aid workers grow to understand and accept the limits of their work, well aware of how small their projects seem in the big scheme of things – a few tiny clinics in a war-ravaged country, a single feeding center in the midst of a famine, a drug distribution program in a tuberculosis pandemic. It's rare for a returning volunteer to rave about how successful her mission was – more often she'll grudgingly admit they helped a few people, saved a few lives. "I felt useless," says nurse Carol McCormack, who worked in a war zone in Burundi. "I didn't change a thing. A few little things, maybe. Acute problems. But I couldn't change those health centers in the time I was there."

It's not just false modesty; it's genuine frustration. Rather than sleeping well knowing they're doing good, aid workers are more likely to be kept awake by what's left to do. "I have people say to me, 'Oh, you work for MSF, that's so noble,'" says one, who reacts to that notion by flipping the bird. "Seriously, you have no idea. It's not noble; it's an *attempt*. People say, 'You must feel so good at the end of the day,' and I'm like, 'Jesus Christ, do you know what happened today?'" That's why so many veterans insist they're not being selfless. As they see it, it's easier to be in the field, getting their hands dirty, feeling involved, than it is to be sitting at home watching the world's crises unfold on TV. And, after that first mission has opened their eyes, sticking their heads in the sand is no longer an option.

Peter Lorber, who did several stints as a logistician, had a profound ambivalence during his tenure, hating many of the things he saw but drawn inexorably back into the lifestyle. "When I was working missions, I really felt alive," he says. "The highs are really high; the horrible things are really horrible. It's not a humdrum life. Even in parts of the missions that are very boring, there are rare, special things that you get so much out of.

"I was in Nigeria when MSF received the Nobel and had a fun time at a quiet reception in the French ambassador's residence. We brought a bunch of local women who were working on our Lagos slum program – I loved watching them camp out next to the buffet, clean off one chicken leg after another, and toss the bones on the carpet. I had the opportunity to eat pepper soup and pounded yam, to drink palm wine and *ogogoro* [a local gin], to get malaria twice. Nigeria is about corruption elevated to a national pastime, sizzling late-night dance clubs, fierce national pride, unimaginably vast oceans of poverty, crime and suffering dotted with islands of obscene luxury and wealth for the fortunate few, mile after mile of windblown trash caught in branches and barbed wire. God, I hated Nigeria. God, I'd love to go back."

After leaving MSF in 2002, Lorber has struggled to feel that vibrancy again. "I don't think I'll ever live like I lived when I was in MSF, including the awful stuff. When MSFers get together at the end of the night and have a party, it's really the best of times. Hard-working people who are crying, getting drunk together afterward. That's really living."

Certainly one of the biggest motivators is the opportunity to visit remote places and experience other cultures. Vincent Echave recalls taking a break from his surgical work in Rwanda and going into the mountains, where he came face to face with a family of gorillas. "There were babies trying to play with my tennis shoes. The male was so big when he stood up, it was unbelievable. What struck me was that I was seeing so much brutality in the cities – in Ruhengeri people were killing each other – and this gorilla was so peaceful." In northern Sri Lanka he watched Tamil villagers walking on fire, and experienced the most bizarre incident that's ever happened on his rounds. "There was a man in the hospital saying he had this pain in his belly. I started talking to him, and he told me he was a snake charmer. I said, 'Oh, that's very interesting, it must be a dangerous profession. Who's taking care of your snake now that you're here, your wife?' And he said, 'No, no, the snake is under the bed.' He got out of the bed and pulled out a basket with some clothes on top, and then he took out a flute, and this king cobra came out of the basket. He started playing with the cobra right in the ward in front of everybody."

Even when those cultures are confounding, there are moments of magic. When nurse Christine Nadori worked in South Sudan – which many MSFers say is close to being on another planet – she remembers running a feeding center among the Dinka, whose culture is centered around their cattle herds. "They don't even tell time in a lot of ways. And you're trying to run a therapeutic feeding program for three hundred to six hundred kids, trying to teach a group of Dinka staff to schedule six milk feedings per day and dole it out in a calculated way to every kid. You lose your mind. But at the end of the day, the sun is going down, the fires are sparking up, a long day closes and the heat starts to abate, women are lining up to get their rations for their kids, the light is gorgeous, and you're laughing. That's when the fun begins."

There are dozens of reasons people go on mission with aid agencies, and some are the wrong ones. Michael Maren, in an interview following the publication of his book, *The Road to Hell*, pulled no punches when asked about the people this work can attract. "There are some really good people out there doing aid work, but I have to say – and this mostly comes from experience as a journalist – that without a doubt, some of the most sanctimonious assholes I have ever met in my life, some of the worst people, and I mean really bad people, work for charities and aid organizations on the ground ... You walk in there and you have life-and-death power over people's lives. And all of a sudden you have a twenty-two-year-old aid worker telling twelve thousand refugees to get over here, to get in line. It gives you a real sense of power."

Maren wasn't talking about MSF specifically, but no organization has a flawless recruiting record. Like any agency that sends its volunteers to far-flung places and gives them a lot of responsibility, MSF has hired expats with colonialist attitudes who have abused national staff, misfits who will never be comfortable in their home societies, and those simply looking for a refuge from problems at home. One head of mission jokes that whenever a new volunteer arrives, she asks, "So, what are *you* running from?"

MSF is wary about its cowboy image, which persists in the aid community, despite the organization's claim that it has outgrown it. "We're very careful not to recruit the Rambos, as we call them – the people who want to do war tourism and catch bullets," says a recruiter. "Those people are the most dangerous of all to a team. If you get a sense that someone's going into this for kicks, that's really not the kind of person you want." MSF's human resources staff also looks for people with more than one language – French or English is essential, since one or the other is the lingua franca in the field – as well as experience working or traveling in developing countries. ("Don't tell us if you did Club Med, because that doesn't count.") Volunteers need flexible lifestyles, since they may be asked to leave for weeks or months on short notice.

MSF also wants people who can work in small groups. "What makes or breaks a mission is the team you're with," says Patrick Lemieux. "You could be in a wonderful country, doing wonderful work, but if you're with a shitty team, you don't have any fun. Or you can be stuck in a compound, not able to stick a finger out, but be with an excellent gang of people and you enjoy your mission."

It's impossible to predict how people will react in the field, however. Teams can include as few as two expats or more than a dozen, and the environments range from quiet villages to all-out conflict, from hot water and cold beer to sleeping on the floor with rats. A logistician who was in South Sudan during a famine spent his first three months living in a tent that was half-submerged in a swamp and infested with mosquitoes. "There had been a long period of dry spells, which had caused the famine, followed by heavy rains," he explains. "We had our living compound on one patch of ground, the supplementary feeding center on another, and then about twenty minutes' walk away was the therapeutic feeding center. During the height of the rainy season we were wading through chest-deep water to get there. You were always wet, you were always cold." It wasn't until after they built a new compound on dry ground, however, that the friction got to them. "After those first three months, I can honestly say there were *more* grumpy people. When the conditions are worst, your team jells much better. You actually have more team-dynamic problems in programs that have been running for a while. Then you have those personality clashes that are a problem in all NGOs."

Nothing brings team members closer together than having the living daylights scared out of them. While Carol McCormack was in Burundi, the town was hit with a mortar attack, leaving her and two young female doctors huddled in the hallway of their house. "It made the bond stronger because we had shared something like that," she says. "We were three people who might not have been friends in another situation – we have nothing in common, and they're both a lot younger than me. They were twenty-eight, and I was thirty-nine. When you're living in very close proximity, and you're stressed, and you're working too hard, and security is bad, there can be spats and difficult times. But then you break loose, and you go and dance your little heart out until two a.m." Often the friendships happen quickly, since there's little time for the rituals of drawing people out of their shell and into the fold. "The pressure is on when you arrive in the team," jokes an administrator with seven missions under his belt. "You better show that you can hang now. Either you drink a beer with us, or you don't. If you don't, you're branded for life."

Before sending volunteers on a first mission, MSF puts its rookies through a training program to introduce them to the organization's philosophy and teach them practical skills, such as how to use a VHF radio or change a tire on a Land Cruiser. (It's also an opportunity for would-be volunteers to bail out if they're having second thoughts.) Much of this prep course focuses on getting along in the field. Nurse Kathleen Bochsler did hers in Amsterdam before heading to Afghanistan. On her first night, she and the other first-timers found themselves in the middle of a Dutch forest at 10 o'clock at night. "They divided us up into groups and gave us maps. Then they piled us into a Land Cruiser, took us out into the woods, dropped us off, and gave us a big tarp and some wooden poles. They said, 'OK, good luck. You have to find this red dot on the map and build a latrine there. We're not telling you where you are, but here's a compass.' Five o'clock in the morning was when this whole fiasco ended. We had found our red dot, built our latrine. The whole time you're learning how to communicate by radio. Of course, they haven't taught you how to communicate before this; they've just given you an idea how frustrating it might be in the field trying to reach somebody.

"At the time, we didn't have any clue what the purpose was. It was just long and brutal, and we were suffering from jet lag.

The next day, you sit down and talk about group dynamics, what problems you had, how you solved them, and what role you felt you played. And that was the most valuable part of the activity, because you're stuck with strangers, you're tired, you're cranky, and you haven't actually made friendships yet. In a lot of ways it's like being on a mission, because you do have to solve problems with people who have totally different ideas. In an organization like MSF, you have a lot of people who are used to being leaders. You throw a bunch of leaders into a group and it's usually chaos."

If there are frequent fights on mission, there's also a lot of making up. Inside jokes about what the initials MSF really stand for range from Meses Sin Follar – Spanish for Months Without Fucking – to the less colorful but more accurate Many Single Females. Take a group of mostly young, strong-minded, unattached people and drop them into an emotionally charged setting far from home, and you've got a recipe for matchmaking. But it's not just opportunity and fewer consequences that bring so many MSFers together. Amid the flings, one-night stands, and missions shortened by pregnancy, long-term relationships form, often lasting for years or for life.

"It's not just that you have a bunch of like-minded individuals, because people join for a thousand different reasons," says Canadian nurse Leanne Olson, who's married to Rink de Lange, a Dutch logistician she met in Bosnia in 1994. "You've got people with different languages and different cultures. There are so many differences it really shouldn't work. But there's an overriding passion for this job among the people who take it seriously, who aren't looking on it as a paid vacation or just an adventure. If you legitimately put something of yourself into the work you're doing, you end up seeing people at their most vulnerable." Olson and de Lange did several missions together and saw each other at their best and worst. "When things go bad, you really see how someone's going to behave. You get to know a person far better, in a short time. You might have friends for years and never really know them, because you've never seen them under pressure, under the stress of these situations. How often in real life are you in a hostage situation or at a dangerous checkpoint with a gun to your head? How often do you see someone get shot in front of you or witness a massacre? With MSF, something along those lines happens in every mission. And then you see how the people on your team react to that. Do they fall apart or do they get closer together? You get to see this aspect of a person's character that's very raw. That's when you see what this person is really going to be like. It makes the process much faster. There's none of this 'Let's date for six months and go out for dinner.'

"I don't have to worry, because one day, if I have a crisis in my life, I know exactly how he's going to behave. With MSF, you know before you ever put on a ring and say 'I do.' I don't have to explain to Rink why I'm watching coverage of the war in Iraq and bawling my eyes out. I don't have to explain to him why, in the middle of a beautiful afternoon in Toronto, when there's an African band playing and everybody's dancing, I'm standing there crying. I don't have to waste any time saying, 'It reminds me of ...'

"You're in that same little boat, and that's where you stay."

4 | Doc in a Hard Place

"This man stepped on an anti-personnel mine," says surgeon Wei Cheng, pointing to the image that fills his computer screen. The patient's tibia and fibula are almost stripped clean of tissue, the bones ending abruptly where the ankle used to be. What remains of the foot hangs by a tenuous ribbon of skin and muscle.

As Cheng moves through the brutal images – just some of 3,000 digital photos that bear witness to the atrocities he saw during his eight months in Kuito, in central Angola – he explains the array of injuries he treated. The civil war was in full swing then, but the bulk of his patients, like the soon-to-be amputee on his monitor now, were not soldiers. Kuito was one of the world's most heavily mined cities, with thousands of land mines lurking on farmland and near water sources, indiscriminately claiming the lives and limbs of civilians.

Cheng arrived in Kuito in the late summer of 2000, along with his Australian wife, Karin Moorhouse, who handled the

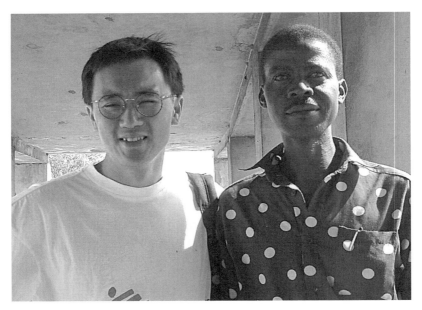

MSF surgeon Wei Cheng and Manuel Vitangui, a nurse in charge of the orthopedic department at the hospital in Kuito, Angola. In November 2000, after soldiers attacked a family in the town, Vitangui went to retrieve the wounded and was killed when his vehicle was ambushed.

project's financial administration. In January 1997, seven months before her death, Princess Diana put Kuito in the world news when she visited the city and dressed in the protective armor of a mine-removal expert for a photograph. By the time Cheng and Moorhouse arrived, an uneasy peace had dissolved and Angola was once again at war. MSF set up a feeding center for the malnourished population, a water and sanitation project for displaced people in a nearby camp, and a hospital program, where Cheng worked with scalpel, saw and suture on thousands of victims of the conflict.

Today, MSF T-shirts are more likely to be seen in less dramatic projects, which often benefit more people or save more lives. But none have a higher profile than surgery in a war zone. "For me," says one physician, "being on the front lines, going into zones that are insecure, trying to provide health care for people who otherwise would not have it – that's the way I've always imagined MSF. It's the whole ambience, too – curfew at five o'clock, gunfire at night. For me, that's MSF. We are where no one wants to be."

Delivering life-saving aid in war zones is at the root of the organization's ethos. Bernard Kouchner and his compatriot physicians in Biafra were part of what came to be called the French Doctors movement, and MSF was born from that initiative. At the time, the Red Cross was the only impartial organization devoted to medical humanitarian aid, but the idea itself arose in an era when wars were fought with bayonets, muskets and cannons and surgeons doubled as barbers. And here, again, there were French doctors.

In 1792, in the wake of the French Revolution, a 26-year-old physician named Dominique Larrey joined Napoleon's army on the Rhine. As assistant surgeon to the French army, he quickly established himself as a pioneer in war medicine. Frustrated that he was watching men die from wounds that had gone untreated for days, he searched for ways to move soldiers quickly from the battlefield to military hospitals and to treat them en route. His solution – the *ambulance volante*, or flying ambulance – was a horse-drawn wagon that rumbled into battle with first-aid supplies, a medical team and their assistants, and a drummer boy who carried the bandages.

Between 1798 and 1815, Larrey took part in just about all of Napoleon's major campaigns, and along the way he became an expert in what we today call emergency medicine. His *ambulance volante* was soon widely used, as was his method of triage

– a previously unknown practice in which medics were trained to identify not only who was the most seriously injured but who had a realistic chance of survival. Just as paramedics do today, Larrey's disciples learned to stabilize the wounded and provide basic treatment in the back of the ambulance as it bounced to the hospital.

Larrey was an innovator in other ways, too. He studied infectious disease outbreaks and learned to quarantine the sick. He performed hundreds of amputations – including 200 in one day during the Battle of Borodino in September 1812 – and his name is still attached to the operation used to remove the arm at the shoulder joint. His preferred anesthetic was a hit of brandy and a cloth to bite down on, although in the freezer of Russia he also learned how cold could be used to numb pain. Just as important as his surgical innovations was his approach to practicing medicine with impartiality. After saving from execution soldiers who were thought to have wounded themselves to escape the fighting, he wrote: "It is not up to the surgeon to determine whether a wound is self-inflicted. That role belongs to a judge. A doctor must be his patient's friend. He must look after both the guilty and the innocent and concentrate his efforts solely on the injury. The rest is not his business." These could have been the words of an MSF doctor two centuries later.

Larrey was a military surgeon and would hardly be called a humanitarian in today's parlance. But because he treated soldiers in any uniform, he gained respect even among France's enemies. During the Battle of Waterloo in 1815, Wellington doffed his hat after spotting Larrey, then turned to an aide and said, "Tell them not to fire in that direction; at least let us give the brave man time to gather up the wounded." This respect eventually saved the doctor's life. After Larrey was shot at Waterloo, he was captured by Prussian soldiers who wanted to execute him. But their field marshal, Gebhard von Blücher, recognized him as the surgeon who, years earlier, had saved the life of his son, when the lad had been wounded in battle. The marshal appointed a Prussian escort to take Larrey safely home to France.

In the photos Wei Cheng and Karin Moorhouse took in Kuito, the city appears as a once-beautiful provincial capital, the buildings now pockmarked with bullet holes. The church and many other structures are without a roof, and some are collapsed completely, though the rubble has been cleaned up. "The city was totally destroyed, yet immaculate," Moorhouse says. "People still had a sense of pride about their city and were out cleaning the streets." The couple has a trio of miniature jeeps, exquisitely fashioned by Kuito's resourceful kids using metal from ration tins, with oil-can stoppers for wheels. Cheng has also kept a clear plastic sandwich bag filled with the bullets he removed from his patients.

The illnesses and wounds Cheng confronted in his operating theater pushed his skills to the limit: a man with deep machete wounds on the side of his face, designed not to kill but to send a warning; a woman with necrotizing fasciitis – flesh-eating bacteria – so advanced that her breast was virtually rotting away; a man with an upper-arm wound crawling with parasitic worms; another with a stab wound four days old, with a section of bowel hanging out. "I pushed it back in, stitched it up, and three or four days later he went home."

Cheng clicks to the next photo, a man whose leg is infected with gas gangrene, an often fatal bacteria that produces gas under the skin, giving it a crackly texture like bubble paper. The surgeon removed the leg just below the hip and pumped the patient with three or four times the normal dose of penicillin. "A week later he was smiling."

Then there are the children. A baby shot through the jaw; an older child with bullet wounds in the shoulder and hand, inflicted deliberately at close range. In another image, a boy about 12 years old holds up a freshly bandaged left hand, still red with blood. "This boy was trying to earn some money by selling things on the street when a policeman asked him for money," Cheng explains. "He didn't give him the money, so the policeman put a bullet through his hand. I couldn't save it." With others, he had better luck. One day a father arrived after carrying his daughter almost 20 miles. She was pale, panting and showing signs of shock, having been shot through the chest, the bullet exiting through the upper back. The father would not allow a blood transfusion, yet she managed to survive.

In November, the bullets struck closer to home. Soldiers, in town looking for women to rape, entered a house and shot a mother and two of her children, including an infant. The father picked up the baby and ran to the hospital, and nurse Manuel Vitangui was sent out to fetch the other wounded. When he arrived, the soldiers ambushed the ambulance and shot Vitangui. "I was in the operating theater trying to rescue the baby when they came in and told me our colleague had been shot. I tried to finish the operation as quickly as possible, but by the time I was done he was already dead."

In all, Cheng did scores of amputations in Kuito, performed with a wire saw. He usually delegated that part of the

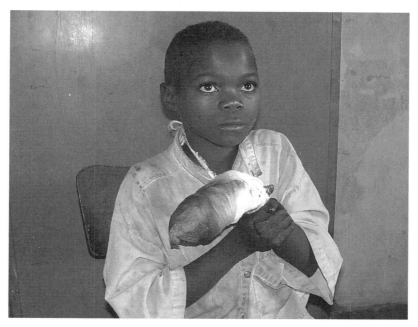

When this boy had no money to pay off police in wartorn Kuito, an officer fired a bullet into the child's left hand, which had to be amputated. During his eight-month mission in Kuito, Wei Cheng performed well over a hundred amputations because of landmine, gunshot and machete wounds.

procedure to one of his assistants because he has no taste for such destruction. Many of his patients were able to take advantage of a nearby prosthesis clinic run by the Red Cross, which fitted them with artificial legs. Cheng later met a German surgeon who spent years in Sierra Leone, where thousands have lost their hands to machete-wielding rebels. This doctor had mastered the Krukenberg procedure, a technique from World War I that leaves the ulna and radius separated, creating a lobster-like claw. This operation is not popular in the West, where it's deemed unsightly and where prosthetic hands are readily available, but in Sierra Leone it's allowed maimed people to lead productive lives.

For a healer, all of this can take a psychological toll. On the day Cheng did his hundredth amputation in Kuito, he and Moorhouse went on a field trip with Halo Trust, the British demining organization that had hosted Diana four years before. "You just stop seeing what's around you," says Moorhouse. "All this becomes so normal. Looking back now, we must have had rocks in our heads."

To reduce the expat turnover all aid organizations face, MSF asks first-time volunteers like Cheng and Moorhouse to commit to at least six months in the field. Surgeons are one exception to that rule, however, not only because it's hard to recruit them for that length of time but because some projects threaten to burn them out in a matter of weeks. In December 2002, MSF rang up American surgeon Bruce Frank, who had done several short missions before, and asked him if he'd like to spend Christmas in Ivory Coast. "They were strapped, and they didn't have anyone who spoke French, but they knew I was trying to learn, so they took a chance and sent me over there. It was quite interesting – I would take a big blackboard into surgery and write down French and English words. It was a struggle at first, and it became a bit comical. They finally told me I was speaking Tarzan French, and that's how I got by. But when it's an emergency and you really need something badly, the whole thing fails you, so there were some touchy moments."

Frank arrived in Abidjan, the Ivorian capital, then drove six hours north to the city of Bouake. "You crossed the ceasefire line that the French soldiers were just implementing there, and someone would pick you up and drive you to the hospital. Bouake is quite a large place – four- or five-hundred-thousand people – but I never really got outside the hospital compound for more than a half-hour the whole time I was there." Though a bustling city in peacetime, some two-thirds of Bouake had emptied out in the previous four months. "MSF sort of took over this hospital, administered it and paid the people, because when the fighting broke out most everybody fled – physicians, nurses and patients as well. There were just eight of us for this huge hospital.

"Everybody was quite ragged the whole time, it was just nonstop," says Frank. "We never did any elective surgery, it was only emergency stuff, and it was 24/7. In five weeks, I had forty or fifty Kalashnikov injuries, plus all the high-speed automotive accidents. Teenagers were walking around with guns – you'd have to walk through a gauntlet of them at the hospital, and you didn't know whether the safety was on or off. I got paranoid about being shot, because I was treating so many gunshot wounds, and many of them were stupid accidental shootings – people getting drunk and shooting their guns, and someone getting hit. I asked why were we tolerating these people being so close to the hospital with their Kalashnikovs – they'd even come into the hospital with them. But it was so busy that we didn't try to do much. We were just on the verge of chaos, and for the first time on any of my missions we lost people I think we shouldn't have lost, just because we were overwhelmed."

One of those was a man about 20 years old who arrived with massive liver trauma. Frank says surgeons back home might see only a couple such injuries in their lifetime. In Ivory Coast, he had one a week. This patient was in danger of bleeding to death and, with no blood available for transfusions, Frank did exactly what a surgeon should. "Instead of trying to repair the liver, I decided just to pack the wound with gauze and close him up. A day or two later, I brought him back in, opened his belly up, took out the packing and repaired the liver. I was quite proud of myself – it was a textbook description of how you should handle a massively damaged liver. Everything looked smooth and wonderful. Then I found out he was still anemic, and on the surgery floor afterward he had a very high heart rate, his blood was still very low. This kid had three friends around him, so I said to them, 'If you don't get blood for him, he's going to die.' They all agreed that they would donate blood. As it turned out, they went to get checked and two of the three were HIV-positive. I was absolutely deflated. The kid died that night, just because of the lack of a couple units of blood.

"In another case, we had a man who was in an auto accident and his liver was shattered, he had a busted femur, and he was in shock. I rushed him to surgery and opened him up, but there was no one around to help me. Finally, they sent in the guy who mops up the floor after surgery. It was incredibly frustrating, because he obviously couldn't help, and the patient ended up dying on the table.

"Toward the end of my mission, there was a child maybe a year old, and no one knew what was wrong with him. We had just finished a twelve- or fourteen-case day, and everybody was tired. We only had one crew of Ivorians – there was no afternoon shift that came on at four o'clock – so we had to be careful not to overschedule them, too, or we'd be shooting ourselves in the foot. At the end of the long day, I went to see this kid, who obviously needed an operation. We talked it over with the other doctors and decided, if the kid is alive tomorrow, we'll do something, because I wasn't sure he'd survive the operation. By this time it was almost midnight, and sure enough, three or four hours later the kid was declared dead. In other circumstances we would have just operated on him. Whether he would have survived, I don't know.

"When I got home, people would ask me how it was, and I would just say it was incredibly intense. I never had to experience a month like that in my life. It just went on endlessly, day and night. General surgery training is famous for 120-hour weeks, every other night on call, but this was every day on call without relief, no backup, no blood, just the basics – and on top of that, the language barrier. Other things begin to wear on you as well – the food, the lack of sleep, the noise when you're trying to sleep. You end up being pretty ragged, and you're not as good as you could be. That's why I've always limited my missions to three or four months, because after that I need to get back to my own reality for a while."

Faced with an overwhelming stream of wounded, Bruce Frank saw just how fine a line separated those who lived from those who died. "You felt that Darwin was part of our triage," he says. When general surgeon Gary Myers made his second trip to Sri Lanka in 2002, he too learned that triumphs and failures can come just days apart. "This was really deep in rebel territory," Myers says of his mission in Point Pedro, at the northern tip of the island nation. "We were taking care of a Tamil population at a hospital, in an isolated community that had been embargoed for something like fifteen years, so they were really lacking medical care. And the area had been heavily mined."

Sri Lanka has one of the highest rates of attempted suicide in the world. "They get trapped in these arranged marriages, and they'll get into fights, and the girl will pour kerosene on herself and set herself on fire. One girl came in with a real dramatic burn – something like sixty percent burned, disfiguring on her face – and over a period of about three weeks, we skin-grafted her ten or twelve times, did lots of wound care, and got a pretty good result. And she was grateful to live. You always worry about that with attempted suicide – if you help them recover just so they can lead a miserable life or try to kill themselves again. Then, within three days, it was kind of the same story – the guy had been drunk, but I think it was a marital spat, and he set himself on fire. But he didn't survive after two or three days. He just couldn't sustain all the stuff we had to do to him."

In July 2003, Myers did a month-long emergency mission in Monrovia, a few weeks after Liberia's civil war returned to the capital. The welcome wagon was there to greet him. "I get there, and I've got my bags and I'm getting my little debriefing, and they come in and say, 'Can you do a tracheostomy on someone?' So I said sure, and there's this guy who had been shot in the neck, and I did a tracheostomy within the first ten minutes I was there.

"In the first two weeks, it was probably eighty-five percent trauma – half of those gunshot wounds and half mortar injuries. One that I'm most proud of was about three days into it. A fifteen-year-old kid got shot in the chest, so we took him to the operating room and opened him up, and he was shot through the heart. We fixed it and he recovered. That's one of those crowd pleasers, but it's not a testament to a good surgeon, that's just good luck. The nice thing about it, though, was it established me with the staff – they thought I was a shaman or something. It was a fortuitous thing to happen early on, because everyone had confidence in me. But the world is a rational place. The next day a guy came in with his abdominal wall blown off from a mortar. I operated on him for three or four hours, and he bled to death. I looked over my shoulder and said, 'Yeah, I'm really not a shaman.'"

In underequipped hospitals like those in Sri Lanka and Liberia, Myers was forced to rely not on tools but on experience. "I'm almost fifty years old, and there are things that I did twenty years ago in the United States that worked pretty well and that didn't require lots of technology. This is one of the criticisms of North American medicine – we've outsmarted ourselves with technology. You can still take pretty good care of a patient without a lot of these things. That's the advantage of a fifty-year-old guy versus a young pup who's twenty-five or thirty. But confidence is not a function of time and experience. I've discovered in my life that I have cycles – sometimes you're very confident and sometimes you get humbled. The neat thing about medicine is you get to go through those things weekly, where you go, 'Boy, I'm an idiot,' or, 'Gosh, I'm right next to Jesus.'"

For a couple of weeks in Liberia, Myers crossed paths with Andrew Schechtman, who was doing his second mission in the country. In the late summer of 2002, Schechtman worked in Harper, a coastal town near the border with Ivory Coast. The catalog of illnesses he tended to drew on every ounce of his training in tropical medicine – rabies, cerebral malaria, elephantiasis, river blindness, not to mention the unpredictable ones, like the young boy who died when a coconut struck him in the head. But even that didn't prepare him for what he faced in the capital. "In Monrovia, when I was in the midst of the fighting, I was definitely more overwhelmed by the needs I wasn't able to meet. I realized in Harper that even doing our best was not adequate, but it didn't slap me in the face. I didn't have three kids a day dying there."

In Monrovia, one of his patients was an 18-month-old girl who was taking a nap when she awoke with a shriek. Schechtman examined the baby and discovered the cause – she had been hit in the cheek with a falling bullet from an AK-47, probably fired randomly into the air by a child soldier. Miraculously, the bullet missed her airway and large arteries.

Several times, random bullets whizzed through the hospital compound, one breaking through the emergency department window, one striking the MSF car, another landing on the kitchen table. Schechtman wondered whether an artillery shell would pay them a house call, too. "There had been a little bit of chronic fighting going on – you'd hear a mortar land in the distance, or in the ocean behind our hospital, with a dull thud. We were getting a steady trickle of patients coming in with wounds from stray bullets, or maybe coming from another part of town where the mortar attacks were heavy – some being brought in by people in a wheelbarrow, or on a stretcher.

"Then suddenly, the mortar attacks were getting louder and closer – we would feel things shaking instead of just hearing the explosion. They would come twenty or thirty seconds apart. Less than five minutes after the mortars got close, people would just start pouring into the emergency room, which had eight beds. The first time we got a big influx of wounded we weren't all that well prepared. Everybody was running around. The nurses, the cleaners, the guys doing the sterilization, everybody was trying to help, which was good, but not very efficient. About seventy people arrived, most of them not life-threatening injuries – they had lacerations, or maybe embedded shrapnel that needed to be treated, but they were not about to die. So for those people we would just slap on a piece of gauze and send them to the next room. A lot of them would just get a ten-second triage and then be shuffled off.

"We had a few people die in the emergency room as soon as they came in. Within a couple of hours, things quieted down and we were able to put a convoy together and send seven or eight of the most severely wounded to the war surgery unit at the Red Cross, about thirty minutes away. Then for the next fifteen hours or so we just started working through this backlog of people, cleaning out wounds, digging out shrapnel, giving tetanus prophylaxis injections." Schechtman knew he had to clear out the patients who were not seriously hurt. "Of course, no one wanted to go home, because these people were living in displaced shelters – abandoned schools, churches, warehouses – with no water, no electricity, not even much shelter from the rain. But I knew that at any time we could get another mortar attack."

The MSF team waited out the shelling in its bunker – a room in their house reinforced with sandbags and with tape on the windows. Like all expats working in war-ravaged countries, they had an escape route in case things got really bad. During one period, Schechtman and his colleagues evacuated to Abidjan, where they discussed whether to abandon the project altogether. When security gets dodgy, MSF headquarters in Europe, or the head of mission in the field, can order an expat team to evacuate, but the volunteers themselves are given leeway to determine how much personal risk they're willing to take. "We knew security was going to be much worse than anything we had dealt with before, with the fighting coming into the town," Schechtman says. "But pretty much all of us decided that we wanted to go back and work in the war zone. And it was clearly the right decision. During those mortar attacks you're seeing kids who are injured, and terrified, and screaming, and you realize that if MSF wasn't there, they would be screaming in the middle of the street with no one to help them."

Christine Nadori has worked in more than a dozen countries with MSF, but only one involved war surgery. She was in Chechnya in 1995, during the early months of the ongoing conflict between Chechens and the Russian army. One evening, as the team was leaving the hospital, Nadori gave the local driver permission to take some of the national staff home. "We were in our house, and we were watching the sun set, and all of a sudden we could hear noise. I thought, oh God, they're not back yet. What's going on? Where are they? I was worried about them, and I shouldn't have let the car go – it was our only car.

"Then I saw this kind of *Apocalypse Now* thing, with these helicopter gunships coming over the ridge. I was really terrified, thinking that our team is on the road and they might target them, but they didn't." In fact, the helicopters were returning from an attack on the town where the MSF driver had dropped off the staff, only a couple of miles away. The bombs began to fall just as the car was leaving. Nadori knew that the wounded would soon be arriving.

"We went to the hospital, and now it was dark, so it was just chaos. People had run to the hospital, and it was full everywhere. We were jumping over people and trying to figure out who were patients, who were wounded. I walked into this one room and there was this kid looking at me. The color of her eyes was just arresting – these humongous gray eyes that would stare at you and never blink, because she was in shock. She was wrapped up in a blanket, and it was completely wet, and I realized she was bleeding. Later someone explained to me what had happened." The girl – years later, Nadori remembers her name was Markha – was about 18 months old. She had been clinging to her mother's back, feet dangling, as the woman ran to escape the fighting. An explosion killed the mother and all but blew off both the girl's feet. "She was one of the first patients we operated on that night. We had to amputate one foot; we tried to salvage part of the other. Whoever had to do her dressings afterward had their heart wrenched out every time.

"Amputation was high on the agenda in that mission. Was I in over my head? Yeah, absolutely. We had restarted a hospital there that had been closed due to the total neglect of the Russian government. It was war, and it was a small team – we were only five. You're exhausted at the end of the day. I assisted as a surgical nurse there for the first time – I had never done surgery before."

Although her stint in Chechnya was just three months, Nadori learned fast and was soon training newly arrived expats in things she'd just learned herself. She remembers a Danish nurse watching in awe as Nadori tenaciously fought to light a defective kerosene burner that they used to sterilize the instruments. "I was doing the sterilization at the same time there was surgery going on, and she was thinking, 'I'm never going to be able to do this.' She thought I was mad. But in a week she was doing the same thing. I've done recruitment, so I've tried to alleviate people's fears about being chucked into the deep end without any resources. We don't ask a nurse to be a doctor, or a doctor to be a surgeon, but you do expand your range of what you can do."

During one of their missions together, Leanne Olson and Rink de Lange had at least one experience where, as nurse and

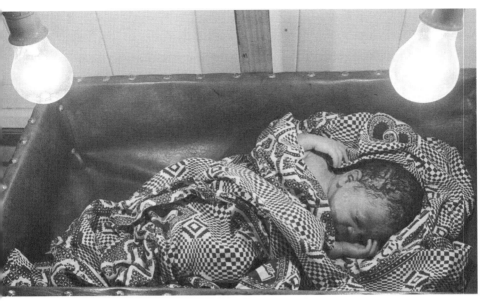

A premature baby is kept warm using an improvised incubator at an Angolan hospital rehabilitated by MSF. Without access to the medical equipment they would use in Western hospitals, expat doctors, nurses and logisticians learn to be resourceful and creative.

logistician, they expanded their job descriptions. "One day we came back from the field, and Valentine, another nurse, said we had a patient," Olson recalls. "We went down to the hospital and this guy had been shot with a machine gun, and he had three bullets in the femur and lower leg. The bullets were still in there, and Valentine said he was going to take them out. I thought, we're going to operate on this guy? We've got no anesthetic, no IV, no medication. And then Valentine said we'd have to put his leg in traction, because his femur was broken. I'm like, 'This is so beyond what I'm capable of doing. We can't do this.' And Rink said, 'Sure we can, we'll think of something.' And we did. Valentine dug the bullets out without even local freezing, in an unsterile situation. I thought for sure the guy was going to bleed to death on the table. Then we put his leg in traction that we had rigged up with rope and ten kilos of stone that we had put in a sack and tied up with tape.

"The guy lived. We took him to the hospital the next day and they're like, 'Hey, nice job with the bullets.'"

5 | In the Yellow Desert

Fifteen miles outside Kandahar, a Land Cruiser rolls effort-lessly along the blacktop. Rugged mountains, not far off but barely visible through the haze, jut sharply from the otherwise pancake-flat landscape. In the back of the vehicle, Dr. Syeed Mahboob Shah shares a bit of local history with the MSF expats – after all, a well-paved highway is so rare in Afghanistan that it begs for an explanation. "It wasn't always like this," says the Afghan physician, smiling under his white baseball cap. "This road was built by the Russians and then destroyed by their own tanks." Only a few years ago you couldn't travel on it, because both sides were strewn with vehicles that had been blown up by anti-tank mines. The Afghans, he says with some pride, have since rebuilt it, cleared the mines and removed their metal casualties.

The pace slows sharply when the driver turns right onto a gravel road. Along both shoulders, oblong concrete markers are painted red on one side, white on the other. "Danger –

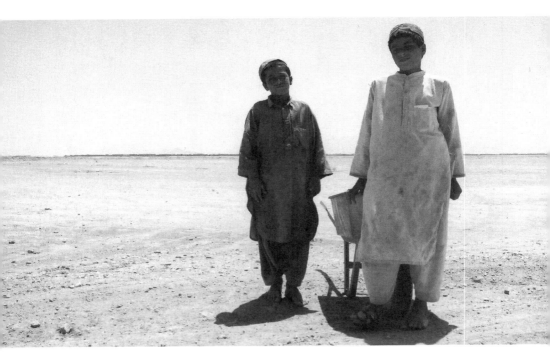

Afghan boys go about their work in the grueling heat and dust of Zhare Dasht, a camp for displaced people in southeastern Afghanistan. MSF operated a basic health unit in the camp until December 2003, when attacks on other aid workers forced them to pull out.

Mines," a sign advises, "Keep Marked Road." Soon a tattered white flag beckons in the distance. Mounted on a bamboo staff, it's emblazoned with the red and black Médecins Sans Frontières logo and marks the entrance of the basic health unit at Zhare Dasht camp for internally displaced people (IDPs). About 40,000 uprooted Afghans make their home in the tents and mud-brick huts of Zhare Dasht, which means "yellow desert" in Pashto. On this day in August 2003, the afternoon temperature hits 111 degrees Fahrenheit. (In winter, it can plummet below zero.) Shade offers some relief, but even indoors it's impossible to escape the dust that squirms its way into the eyes, nose and mouth. Outside, winds twist the sand into towering dust devils.

Many of Zhare Dasht's residents are Pashtuns, the ethnic group that spawned the Taliban. Pashtuns make up much of the south and east of Afghanistan, but since the Taliban fell from power in 2001, Pashtuns have become a persecuted minority in the north, harassed and attacked by vengeful Uzbeks, who dominate that area. Those able to escape to the south have sought protection and aid in camps like Zhare Dasht. The camp's other main group are Kutchis, nomads whose emerald and magenta clothing and beautiful blue-green eyes gleam amid the sea of white, black and khaki favored by Pashtuns. They have not come here to escape war but, rather, the four-year drought that has parched the earth and wiped out their herds.

A Kutchi girl in a pretty pink dress and green headscarf carries her little brother into a tent that functions as a supplementary feeding center. Here children are weighed in a basin that hangs from a scale, and those between 70 and 80 percent of their normal weight are given high-protein food supplements. Inside the feeding center, nurse Kathleen Bochsler is just getting used to the challenges of being a woman in Afghanistan. Bochsler and the other female expats have to keep their heads, legs and arms covered whenever they leave their Kandahar compound. Between her sunglasses and sandals, she's pulled an MSF vest over a blue and white *salwar kameez* – the loose-fitting cotton pants and tunic worn by locals – and topped the motley outfit with a burgundy headscarf. "This is a fashion crisis," she joked before leaving for the camp that morning. "It's more than that," answered her colleague, Hernan del Valle, the resident wit. "It's a humanitarian emergency."

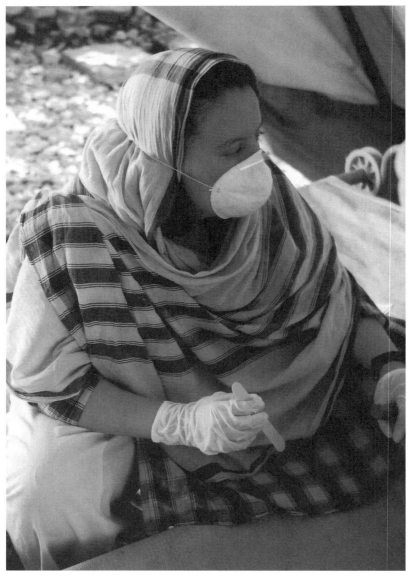

Canadian nurse Kathleen Bochsler examines patients for diphtheria in a tent outside Kandahar's Mir Wais Hospital. After an outbreak in the nearby Zhare Dasht camp, MSF inoculated thousands of displaced people against the potentially deadly infection.

Bochsler, a Canadian who looks younger than her 30 years, is just four weeks into her first mission, but she's no stranger to delivering health care in difficult places. After graduating with her nursing degree, she worked on a Native reserve in northern Ontario, then in a small rural hospital near the British Columbia–Alaska border, and most recently on a reserve in Manitoba with an unsavory reputation. Although MSF looks for volunteers who have worked in developing countries, it appreciates this kind of Canadian experience, too. "It's isolated and you're dealing with not having support services and equipment," Bochsler says. "Patients may have to be flown out, so there's a long delay in care. You have to learn how to manage stress, solve problems. I think they liked me for Afghanistan because I was from a violent reserve, so I was security conscious."

As in many MSF projects, the main responsibility of the expat team here is to assist, train and support the local staff. To be able to do that, the medical team must first understand the cultural context it's working in. The organization runs hundreds of feeding centers around the world, but the one they have set up in Zhare Dasht is unusual, because the camp is relatively well provisioned by the United Nations. "The problem is, when children are sick, they are given only tea," says Bertien van Gijssel, the project's Dutch physician. "You can imagine that if they are given only tea, children can get malnourished." At the feeding center, not only do the kids receive nourishing food, but the staff educates the parents about proper feeding.

Adjusting her headscarf, Bochsler joins Mahboob Shah for a short drive to an area of the camp unimaginatively named Settlement 10. At 6 o'clock that morning, dozens of MSF national staff set up a vaccination center there, and they've spent the day inoculating 1,200 people for diphtheria. It's a disease that neither Bochsler nor van Gijssel had ever seen before – vaccinations have eradicated it from Western countries, and even in developing nations it's a rare ailment that MSF doesn't encounter often. There have been about 50 cases in the camp during the past month, however, and MSF has asked the UN's World Health Organization in Geneva for advice. It's also relying on the Afghan doctors and nurses, who have experience diagnosing and treating it. Caused by a contagious bacterium that inflames the mouth and throat, the disease can produce a toxin that's fatal in about 10 percent of cases. "Diphtheria is a little bit endemic in Kandahar," van Gijssel says, "but the antitoxin has never been in the city itself, so people were always going to Pakistan, or they would die. So the first thing we had to do, together with WHO, was get the antitoxin from Islamabad to Kandahar so we could treat the patients in the hospital. After that, we decided to do a mass vaccination for the whole camp."

When the expats and the national staff have a good working relationship, they exchange information both ways. Van Gijssel says the Afghan doctors and nurses have taught her not just about diphtheria but also about measles, which Western doctors often learn about from pictures in textbooks, not first-hand observation. She says the local medics are largely well trained, with one big blind spot. "During the Taliban, there were only male doctors, and gynecology and obstetrics were taken out, so they know nothing about menstruation, menopause, spontaneous abortion, delivery. They know nothing about STDs, because they have never examined a woman. But they are very eager to learn about it." Even in

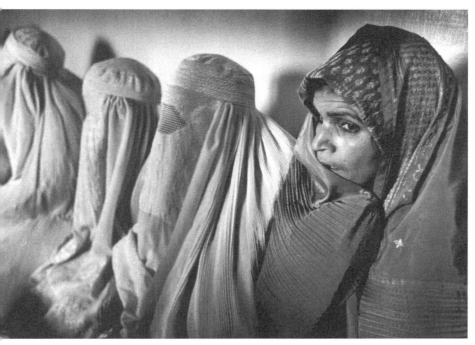

At this clinic in Mazar-e-Sharif, MSF provides education sessions for Afghan women, covering hygiene, breastfeeding and basic health care. Even after the fall of the Taliban, doctors in Afghanistan may have to examine women through a burqa, making diagnosis a unique challenge.

post-Taliban culture, male doctors cannot give females a full examination – they listen to the heart and lungs through clothing, sometimes even through a burqa, the heavy garment that covers the bodies and faces of many Pashtun women. What this means is that doctors have to make guesses, so they tend to overprescribe antibiotics. In other cases, they may underestimate conditions like abdominal pain or gynecological problems because they don't have enough information.

Near the well at Settlement 10, a barefoot boy approaches the car, his face covered in scabs. "It looks like impetigo,"

Bochsler says, "which is very common back home, especially in First Nations communities." Here, she explains, the only treatment she's seen is gentian violet, which is ineffective in advanced cases. "When you see it to that degree at home you'd always put them on oral antibiotics." Here again, delivering health care in Afghanistan means not only having the right drugs but convincing a sometimes reluctant population to use them. Mahboob Shah says that during the diphtheria vaccinations many patients refused the needle. "There are rumors that the vaccine causes infertility." In other cases, though, Afghans have proven fond of injections, which most believe are superior to oral medication – especially white pills, which are considered useless because they all look the same. The rule of thumb when it comes to tablets, says van Gijssel, is "the bigger the better, and the redder the better."

Wars, natural disasters and persecution have driven people to flee their home countries since time immemorial. Even the English word *refugee* is centuries old, first appearing in 1685 and originally referring to the Huguenots who came to England to escape religious persecution. The current legal definition of refugee, however, has been on the books only since 1951, when the Convention Relating to the Status of Refugees was adopted in Geneva and the United Nations High Commissioner for Refugees (UNHCR) was appointed its guardian. Article 1 defines a refugee as "a person who is outside his/her country of nationality or habitual residence; has a well-founded fear of persecution because of his/her race, religion, nationality, membership in a particular social group or political opinion; and is unable or unwilling to avail himself/herself of the protection of that country, or to return there, for fear of persecution." The 1951 agreement was intended to protect and resettle 1.2 million Europeans who had been uprooted during World War II. In 1967, the Protocol Relating to the Status of Refugees widened the geographical scope of refugee law. Today, 145 countries have ratified one or both of these agreements.

None of the convention's 19 original signatories could have anticipated how the world's refugee situation would evolve in the decades to come. As 2003 opened, there were about 10.4 million refugees worldwide, approximately the same number as in 1982, though far fewer than the peak of almost 17.8 million in 1992. UNHCR works to ensure that these refugees receive official status, which entitles them to protection and assistance. If and when circumstances permit, the organization helps them return home and rebuild their lives, but in the meantime one of its roles is to set up and administer camps where refugees can receive shelter, food and medical aid. It's an enormous task that is increasingly subcontracted to government organizations, private companies and international aid agencies like Médecins Sans Frontières. MSF cut its teeth in refugee camps in the late 1970s and early 1980s, and it now brings decades of experience to delivering health care in these environments.

In the months following the US-led attack on the Taliban that began in October 2001, hundreds of thousands of Afghans scattered, some to other parts of the country, others to neighboring Iran and Pakistan. Decades of conflict and years of drought had already pulled the rug out from under Afghanistan, the world's leading exporter of refugees, but this crisis was unprecedented. A little perspective: At the beginning of 2002, there were about 12 million refugees worldwide. Of these, more than 3.8 million – almost a third – were Afghans. Another 1.3 million Afghans were internally displaced. When you consider that the country's population is about 28 million, about that of New York and New Jersey, these numbers are staggering. Between March and November 2002, more than 1.8 million Afghan refugees returned to their country, the largest homecoming in history, and hundreds of thousands have since followed. But millions more are still living in camps both inside and outside Afghanistan, completely reliant on aid agencies.

While the rights of refugees are enshrined in international law, internally displaced people – who may number 25 million worldwide – inhabit a gray area. They are, strictly speaking, the responsibility of their own governments. But because governments often lack the resources or the political will to look after these people, UNHCR has stretched its mandate to include millions of them, including those at Zhare Dasht. Indeed, the Afghan situation is a prime example of how the distinction is in some ways a mere technicality. Within a couple of hours' drive from Zhare Dasht is a network of other camps – one in Spin Boldak, on the Afghan side of the border, and several others near the town of Chaman, Pakistan. Whether refugees or IDPs, the Afghan families in these camps face the same medical predicament that comes from cramped conditions, exposure to a harsh climate, inadequate water and sanitation, and despair.

In several of these camps, and in many others around the world, MSF provides basic health care for months or years and intervenes in acute emergencies, such as outbreaks of disease.

A refugee camp provides ideal conditions for all manner of pestilence. One of the most rampant is measles, which kills almost a million people each year in developing countries, most of them children. Although its most familiar symptom is a distinctive skin rash, measles is a respiratory infection that is caused by an airborne virus transmitted the same way as the common cold – through coughing and sneezing. In an overcrowded refugee camp, where people may already be weakened by inadequate nutrition, measles outbreaks can be swift and deadly. Measles vaccination is priority number one when setting up shop in a refugee camp, and MSF tries to make sure that all the children between the ages of 6 months and 15 years are immunized. These campaigns may also include a vitamin A distribution, since a deficiency of this nutrient can increase the measles mortality rate.

Cholera is another disease that is easily prevented and treated in developed countries. Among refugees and displaced people, however, it can lead to an agonizing death. Caused by a bacteria, *Vibrio cholerae*, cholera is usually transmitted when infected feces comes into contact with the mouth, often with the help of flies, contaminated water, unwashed hands or improvised latrines. Many infected people have no symptoms, but the unfortunate ones suffer vomiting and copious diarrhea – discharging up to a quart of fluid an hour in severe cases. Some patients are so weakened that they have to use a "cholera bed" – a stretcher with a strategically positioned hole, placed over a bucket. Left untreated, cholera can be fatal in up to 50 percent of cases, but a simple course of rehydration, either orally or intravenously, can bring a quick turnabout. Other diarrheal diseases – including those caused by *Shigella* or *E. coli* bacteria – cause even more deaths among displaced people.

Despite the squalor of a refugee camp, life and love go on as before. Some of the 100 to 120 daily visitors to the basic health unit at Zhare Dasht have broken bones or lacerations suffered in minor mishaps; many have respiratory problems or irritated eyes – both largely due to the unmerciful dust. Diarrheal diseases are common, especially in the summer, when the heat allows the bacteria to flourish around the pumps and jerry cans that carry the camp's water supply. Many patients show up with headaches, body pains and other complaints that have a psychosomatic cause, not unusual in a population that has endured years of stress and hardship. The vast majority are treated on the spot or given medication from the camp's pharmacy. The basic health unit also has a nursing station for dressing wounds and performing simple diagnostic tests, a vaccination area for children under 2 and women of childbearing age, and a tent where pregnant women can visit a midwife. There are two consulting doctors – one for men, another for women. Health care, like virtually all activities in Afghanistan, is strictly segregated by sex. Perhaps five or six patients each day are sick enough to have to endure the one-hour drive to Mir Wais Hospital.

On January 8, 2002, in a second-floor ward of Mir Wais Hospital in Kandahar, seven men were crowded into a single room. Nursing three-week-old wounds that had never been properly treated and living on bread, oranges and cookies smuggled in by bribed staff, they were no doubt in considerable agony. One of the seven, apparently unable to endure his hospital stay any longer, shaved his beard to disguise his appearance and tried to make a hasty exit. When he was quickly surrounded by Afghan soldiers, the patient held a grenade to his chest, pulled the pin and checked out for good.

Like his six colleagues, the dead man was an al-Qaeda fighter, one of several who had been dropped off at Mir Wais in December after being wounded in battles with the Americans or their Afghan allies. A few had already escaped from the hospital without being captured, and two others were lured out by a ruse and promptly arrested. Eventually six remained, holed up with some 120 other patients, refusing to surrender even to the Red Cross and vowing they would use their pistols and grenades if their enemies tried to take them alive. Before dawn on January 28, Afghan and US special forces, weary of the siege, surrounded the hospital. After hours of maneuvering, they attacked, lobbing several grenades into the building and then storming the ward. In the firefight that ensued, the last of the al-Qaeda patients were mowed down by assault rifles, some while hiding under their beds.

Nineteen months later, nurse Mohammed Yaqub walks along a freshly painted corridor at Mir Wais, which has been rehabilitated with the help of MSF. One of the most experienced of the national staff on this project, Yaqub has seen many expats come and go as teams have been evacuated and recalled. He's even outlasted the Taliban. His tidy black beard was much longer during their reign, of course – he could have been lashed or jailed for trimming it. "Those were very difficult years," he says, with decided understatement.

MSF is supporting the infectious diseases ward in the renovated hospital, which has become suddenly busy in the wake of the diphtheria outbreak at Zhare Dasht. Because of limited space, patients recovering from the disease are sheltered outside in large tents, where small electric fans are out-matched by the stifling heat. The fact that diphtheria patients are here at all is something MSF had to fight for, says Kathleen Bochsler. When the first reports of diphtheria came in from the camp, the Afghan ministry of public health and the WHO asked MSF to stop referring the patients to Kandahar. "They said it was putting the city at risk for diphtheria, and they didn't want them at the hospital. They said they'd build a little hospital at the camp and we could treat them there. Well, in theory, that's wonderful. But if there's an emergency, like an anaphylactic reaction, they're an hour away from Mir Wais. If it's anaphylaxis, they'll be dead."

Besides, the antitoxin used to treat diphtheria can't be given in extreme heat – the temperature must be below 95 degrees, and at Zhare Dasht the mercury can reach 120. "At least at the hospital, we have fans and water coolers," Bochsler says. At Mir Wais, the 48-hour antitoxin treatment can be given inside the infectious diseases ward, and only then are the patients moved to the recovery tent, where they spend a week on antibiotics. So MSF did what it usually does in these situations: it refused to work on terms it found unacceptable. "We said to the WHO and the ministry of public health, unless you can replicate what we're doing in the city, we are not going to sup-port your building a little hospital in the camp, and we said if they didn't meet certain criteria we wouldn't send our patients there. That made us very unpopular. However, after we put that all in writing and submitted it, they changed their mind." As a rookie, Bochsler admits to being surprised that MSF won this argument. "I'm still trying to get my head around the fact that if we don't agree with something here, we don't do it."

Above the walls of the MSF compound in Kandahar, you can occasionally glimpse a kite flitting about in the dry wind. It's a triumphant gesture, a less contrived version of the Marines raising the US flag at Iwo Jima. Before the Taliban was ousted from this area, kite-flying was outlawed, along with such other vices as music, public laughter and white shoes. The bans on wicked footwear are gone now, but there's still a Taliban presence in and around Kandahar, says Mattias Ohlson as he sits in the inadequate shade a dozen yards from the compound's bunker. The 31-year-old Swede is on his third mission with MSF and, as the project coordinator, it's his job to keep on top of security. The UN and coalition forces are supposed to advise NGOs about any potential dangers, but they don't always keep pace with the word on the street, Ohlson says. "We also send the local staff to the bazaar to talk to taxi drivers and things like that."

Having a close relationship with community leaders and the general population isn't just important for security. "For me, that is one of the reasons to work with MSF," says Bertien van Gijssel. "To go into cultures where no one else goes and see the daily lives of people, to do the work that you love and have a little adventure. And also to see what is really going on in these countries, because you hear a lot, especially from Afghanistan, and it's quite interesting to see how people really live." That's been almost impossible in Kandahar, though, where the MSF team is under virtual house arrest. "Many times we are invited to the homes of national staff, but we can't go because they live on narrow streets and we can't park the cars there. We are not allowed to walk around the streets –

we're always getting into the car inside our compound, and getting out in the compound of another NGO. We've been shopping only once or twice, always accompanied by national staff. At a certain point, you want to go out into the streets and see what's happening or ride a bicycle. You really feel quite locked up."

Van Gijssel was pleased to finally get a peek under the burqas when she was invited to a local wedding. "Of course, the men had to go with the men, and the women had to go to a female party. Then you suddenly see all these women who are totally dressed up – they come in with their burqas, then they take them off and dress up in very nice clothes and start dancing all night long, really enjoying themselves. No scarves, with makeup on. It was amazing. It's such a strange situation, because the men never see the women like this. Unfortunately, we had a curfew and the party was just getting started when we had to go."

By Kandahar standards, the MSF compound, which includes both office and living quarters, is more than comfortable. There's cold running water, a fridge with a few cans of Heineken, some maple syrup for the Canadians. The television gets CNN and the BBC, and there's a video-disc player to screen pirated movies purchased in Pakistan. There's a CD player, too, though music is still hard to find in Afghanistan. ("You can get CDs in Herat now," says Hernan del Valle. "It's the first stage of reconstruction. The second stage is McDonald's. After that comes health care.") An old man even tends a small garden, where Ohlson hopes to plant some vegetables to enliven the menu. The withered pomegranate trees don't inspire confidence, but locals boast that Kandahar still produces grapes "sweet enough to make men cry."

On this day, Ohlson says, the team is worried about a doctor and a nurse coming to Kandahar from the MSF project in Chaman, Pakistan, about two hours to the southeast. Part of a notorious smuggling route that stretches from Iran to India, the road from the Pakistani border to Kandahar may be the most dangerous in Afghanistan. Not long ago, it wasn't unusual to encounter dozens of checkpoints along the 60-mile road, each manned by Kalashnikov-toting warlords demanding a toll. These days it's more likely to be patrolled by American soldiers flushing out the Taliban – many have escaped to Pakistan, but they return occasionally to stir up trouble, and this is their favorite route. Less than three weeks ago, US aircraft attacked an area nearby, killing 24 Taliban fighters. With Afghanistan's independence-day celebrations coming next week, Ohlson is worried there may be another incident.

While the MSF medical team travels in a clearly marked Land Cruiser, red crosses and other humanitarian logos no longer offer protection in this region. In fact, NGOs may as well paint targets on their vehicles these days. Indeed, in Chaman, the MSF team travels in unmarked vans and flies no flag over its compound. No aid worker had been killed in Afghanistan since 1998, but everything changed on March 27, 2003, when Ricardo Munguía, a Salvadoran water engineer with the International Committee of the Red Cross, was stopped with his convoy by armed Taliban in Uruzgan province. According to a witness, the gunmen first poured gasoline on the vehicles and set them alight. Then they called their mullah on a satellite phone to ask for instructions. The reply: Kill the foreigner. The gunmen pumped 20 bullets into Munguía. (To add a cruelly ironic twist, the mullah who ordered Munguía's execution uses an artificial leg provided by the Red Cross.) The compound where Munguía lived is a two-minute drive from the MSF house, and the team often goes there for a party or a dip in what might be the only decent swimming pool in Kandahar.

Several more attacks on aid workers followed. On the very day Ohlson described his security concerns, two members of the Afghan Red Crescent Society were shot by gunmen who fled on motorcycles – a Taliban trademark – in Ghazni province to the north. Three weeks later, five workers with the Danish Committee for Aid to Afghan Refugees were stopped by nine armed men, dragged from their vehicle and tied up. The attackers berated the men for working with an aid organization, then murdered four of them; the fifth miraculously survived. "It's a difficult situation to be in," says Ohlson. "You have to be constantly alert to what is happening in your area and spend lots of time drinking *chai* with different people, who become part of your security network. There is a great deal of uncertainty, and you don't know what tomorrow will bring."

It's little wonder that the MSF compound has a bunker, complete with food, bottled water, a small stove, a VHF radio connection and a satellite phone. David Croft, the logistician on the Kandahar project, is even planning an improvement. "I'm thinking of putting a pickax in there so we can tunnel out if the shit really hits the fan." He and van Gijssel got to try out the bunker just days after arriving. "It was quite good fun in hindsight," Croft says, "though at the time it was a bit scary. Bertien and I showed up in this project and were greeted by just the national staff, who'd been holding it together for three months when the previous expats had been pulled out. Usually you go into a project and you've got three or four expats who take you under their wing. Well, Bertien is second mission and I'm first mission, both of us new to Afghanistan, and neither of us had a clue what was going on. We had a ball when we first came here and didn't really see the big issue about security. We respected it, but we hadn't seen anything yet. Then one day I was sitting in the administration office and a bomb went off down the road at an NGO house – a small grenade or something was thrown over the fence. That was all very exciting."

The next night, it got even more exciting. "We were up in the office doing some e-mailing and *bang* – something went off with such a blast. I've traveled in a lot of dodgy countries before and I've heard explosions, but nothing that big, that close. It didn't blow any windows out, which was surprising because these windows are about as strong as wet cornflakes. Bertien was already down the steps on her way to the bunker. I dove for the switches and started turning off lights, because I'd seen in a movie once where someone did that. I was just running around, not sure what the hell I was doing. We were totally unprepared, no shoes on, nothing. I got the computer and the mini-M [satellite phone] and jumped into the bunker. We phoned the country management team in Herat and they were quite cool, they really calmed us down. Then we smoked a dozen cigarettes each, and it was all pretty good."

Eventually the whole story emerged. The blast turned out to be from an old Chinese-made 107 mm rocket that had misfired – only the fuel exploded, not the business end. Croft believes it was ignited by someone trying to send a warning to the governor, who lives a stone's throw from the MSF house. "So that whole big blast that showered gravel and sand into our compound two doors down was actually nothing more than the fuel going off. I'd hate to see the warhead."

On October 4, 2003, the attacks came to the doorstep of the Zhare Dasht basic health unit. Four armed men, most likely Taliban, entered the outskirts of the camp and rounded up six members of a mine-clearing NGO. They were about to execute them on the spot when one of the agency's drivers started his truck and tried to escape. The gunmen, distracted from their task, turned to shoot at the vehicle, and the deminers ran for their lives. They all managed to escape, though one was shot in the leg. The MSF driver heard the shooting and grabbed the radio to warn other vehicles to stay away. "Kathleen and I were almost in the camp at the moment it happened," van Gijssel remembers, "and we had to turn back without any information – that was quite frightening. We had only heard that there was a car coming toward us, and they said, 'You have to leave, it's not safe, there's shooting, the Taliban is here.' There is only one road in and out of the camp, so you just have to hope that nothing is going to happen."

After the incident, MSF had no choice but to stop its work at Zhare Dasht. "Suspending medical activities is, of course, always a very difficult decision to make," says Ohlson. "In this case, ten thousand families in the camp depend on the health care, and more than two hundred people visit the clinics every day." While the expats stayed in Kandahar, local staff, some of whom live in the camp, set up a triage and ambulance system. "They worked really hard for long hours, treating some of the people and sending the seriously ill ones to the hospital or a clinic closer to the city. We had seven minivans shuttling back and forth."

Within two weeks, Ohlson convinced the governor to provide more checkpoints around the camp and the team returned. By December, however, the situation had deteriorated further, and MSF once again withdrew to Kandahar and confined its work to Mir Wais Hospital.

It was in the northwestern province of Badghis, ironically one of the safer places in Afghanistan, that MSF's luck ran out on June 2, 2004. A Land Cruiser carrying five staff was ambushed by gunmen, believed to be Taliban fighters. Whether words were exchanged or warning was given, no one is ever likely to know, as the team never checked in by radio after setting off around 3 pm. Later that afternoon the car was discovered – it had been shredded by gunfire, and shrapnel indicated a grenade had exploded. It was a heinous murder of five unarmed aid workers: Belgian project coordinator Hélène de Beir, Dutch logistician Willem Kwint, Norwegian doctor Egil Tynaes, their Afghan translator Fasil Ahmad and their driver Besmillah. Just weeks before the slaying, while de Beir was taking a break in Italy, she told a friend, "I am exhausted, physically and emotionally." The friend asked why she was going back. "Because I have to," the 30-year-old replied. "It's what makes me happy."

The next day, MSF suspended its work in Afghanistan and withdrew its teams to Kabul. In Badghis, as in Zhare Dasht, the teams will eventually return, as long as there are patients who need their help. Until then, they'll keep the dust out of their eyes and watch the way the winds blow in the yellow desert.

6 | Ugly Realities

On the day Lloyd Cederstrand's tiny bush plane touched down in a remote area of South Sudan, he watched six children die. He wasn't surprised, then, when other expats decided this MSF mission wasn't for them. "I saw people get off the plane and, twenty-four hours later, they would get back on it. It was overwhelming to come in and see such high mortality rates."

Cederstrand stuck it out for three months as a logistician during the 1998 famine in South Sudan, one of the worst of the decade. Like so many food shortages in Africa, this one was caused by a combination of warfare, drought and economic factors, and it left as many as a quarter of a million people dead from starvation and illness. One of Cederstrand's duties was supervising the food drops that regularly arrived as part of Operation Lifeline Sudan, the huge international relief effort. "It's very dangerous – people have been killed, cattle have been killed, villages have been flattened when they miss the drop zone. An X literally marks the spot – you have a massive

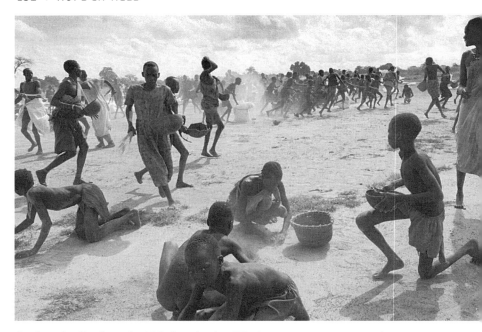

During the famine of 1998, hundreds of Sudanese converge on a drop zone to collect bits of maize. This image was captured by logistician Lloyd Cederstrand, whose tasks included securing the area for the World Food Programme's weekly deliveries by air to MSF's feeding centers in the region.

X made of plastic sheeting. You'll pick your drop zone in the driest area you can find, and then you have a lot of national staff keep the area clear, because as soon as people know a food drop is going to happen they congregate in the area. When the Hercules comes over, it slows down, the back comes open, and the pallets just roll out of the plane and free-fall onto an area about the size of a football field." Cederstrand says only 6 or 7 percent of the bags break, and almost nothing is wasted. "When security lets the people come in, you have thousands converging on the drop zone with their little gourds and their little bowls, scooping up dirt or mud just to get ten pieces of maize."

MSF is not usually involved in general food distribution – that's the domain of the UN's World Food Programme – but in famine-stricken areas it sets up feeding centers to treat malnourished children, pregnant women, nursing mothers and the elderly. At therapeutic feeding centers (TFCs), severely malnourished kids under five stay with a family member and receive feedings of high-protein powdered milk. Supplementary feeding centers provide moderately malnourished children with meals and an extra ration to take home.

There are few sights more heart-rending than a starving child, but those who are admitted to a TFC in time can recover within 30 days. In the critical first phase, the child receives six or more feedings a day of therapeutic milk that includes oils, vitamins and sugar and is designed to kick-start the metabolism. "That will take a few days, and it's a really risky period," says Christine Nadori, who was a nutritional coordinator in South Sudan in 1998. "You might lose some if they're anemic and have a weakened heart – you're increasing their blood volume, and the heart starts going wild. Or they may not have enough hemoglobin left to bring oxygen to the tissue. Usually they spend two or three days in a critical period, where we give them small quantities of milk, based on how much they weigh already, and then we increase it as their muscle mass starts to increase. They may spend a month in a TFC, until they reach a certain weight, and then they'll graduate to a supplementary feeding center." Here they'll receive solid food – porridges, beans, high-protein BP-5 biscuits or Plumpy'nut, a kind of therapeutic peanut brittle.

The feeding centers set up by MSF and other organizations in Sudan saved tens of thousands of lives in 1998. Still, Cederstrand's project forced him to confront one of the limits of humanitarian aid. "For me, it can be overwhelming to be treating someone in a TFC so you can send them out into a situation that you can't change. That child I'm discharging today is probably going to be right back here six months later."

In addition to conflict zones, refugee camps and feeding centers, MSF hangs out its shingle in tiny health outposts in remote communities, in mobile clinics that travel from village to village in a Land Cruiser, and in areas hit by floods, eruptions or other natural disasters.

The first step in most of these projects is an exploratory mission, or explo, which involves sending a small team into an area to assess the medical needs and judge whether an intervention is necessary. These short-term projects measure mortality rates, morbidity rates (the local prevalence of disease) and the level of malnutrition in a population. The medical team may set up sentinel surveys, which monitor the rate of measles, malaria, diarrhea or cholera at selected sites and quickly identify an outbreak when it occurs. An explo will also look at the medical infrastructure to see if the local health ministry has things under control. It will determine whether other NGOs are planning to work in the area. And if MSF decides to intervene, it will find out who is in charge and get permission to work there.

This last point may be one of the most misunderstood aspects of MSF. The *sans frontières* ethos that's enshrined in the organization's name suggests a willingness to ignore sovereignty and governments wherever people are suffering. Even the Nobel committee, when announcing the Peace Prize, commented that a fundamental principle of MSF is that "national boundaries and political circumstances or sympathies must have no influence on who is to receive humanitarian help." In its presentation speech, the committee reiterated that MSF "reserved the right to intervene to help people in need irrespective of prior political approval."

These statements caused some uneasiness among the new Nobel laureates. Joelle Tanguy, then executive director of MSF-USA, said in a November 1999 speech: "At MSF, we have trouble recognizing ourselves as the standard bearers of this 'right to intervene,' which a number of interviews and articles seem to indicate as having been finally acknowledged and sanctioned by the award ... We cannot let such a serious misunderstanding become entrenched." MSF was worried that the line was blurring between the right to deliver medical aid to victims – something enshrined in the Geneva Conventions – and what had taken place in Kosovo earlier that year. As David Rieff writes in *A Bed for the Night*, "many humanitarians supported the war on moral grounds. But just because individual humanitarians and, for that matter, some humanitarian NGOs were for the war, this did not make what took place a *humanitarian intervention*, although that was precisely what major NATO powers tried to claim it to be."

So, what exactly does "without borders" mean to MSF? "It's a very malleable concept which has changed in significance over time," says Austen Davis of MSF-Holland. "In the Cold War, when MSF started in the seventies, it was a provocative statement, saying we're going to help people, and it doesn't matter if they're Communists." The organization entered Afghanistan without the permission of Soviet forces in 1980, and as recently as 2003 it launched a clandestine cross-border mission into southern Iraq, retreating back into Kuwait every evening. But these activities were confined to areas outside the direct control of the Soviet and Iraqi armies, respectively. "Of course you're going to require a yes from whoever is in control of an administrative area," Davis says. "You have to, because they've got guns and they can shoot you otherwise. All we're saying is that if, say, South Sudan is for all intents and purposes, administered by rebels and the government says, 'We don't recognize them, and we are a sovereign state and you have to get your visas from us to go into the south,' we say, 'Nonsense,' and we don't. We will if that helps, but if that is going to be the barrier to helping people, we will not respect that requirement.

"I think *frontière* implies other things as well. In Bunia [in eastern Congo], a town we've had a long relation to, we insist on working with the Hema and Lendu, and both sides tried to stop us working with the other, so that's an ethnic *frontière*. Now it's extremely important for us, somehow, to be able to cross the Christian-Islamic *frontière*. These borders that distinguish people, that allow the demonization of the other – that is, in part, what humanitarianism is against. It is against the dehumanization of people in crisis."

"On the practical level, you do things legally if you can," says Kenny Gluck of MSF-Holland. "Only when it becomes impossible to assist people would you transgress in that way. Being in touch with authorities is one of the foundations of humanitarianism. Unlike charity, humanitarianism doesn't exist in a vacuum, it operates in a dirty reality, and that forces you to struggle with your principles. It's not a pure exercise. *Sans frontières* is a mentality – it's always about engaging with ugly realities so that you can get something done. It's aspirational in

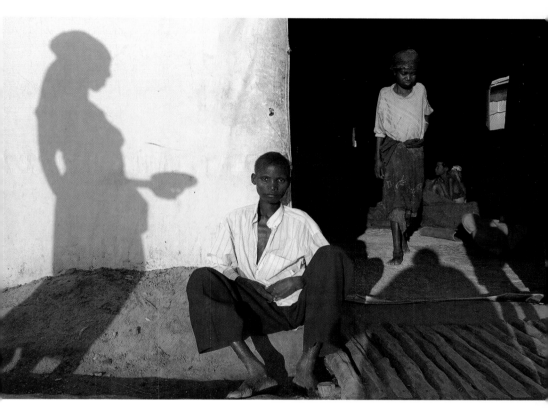

Peace in April 2002 finally allowed humanitarian agencies access to thousands of starving Angolans. MSF quickly set up this therapeutic feeding center in Kuito to treat severely malnourished children.

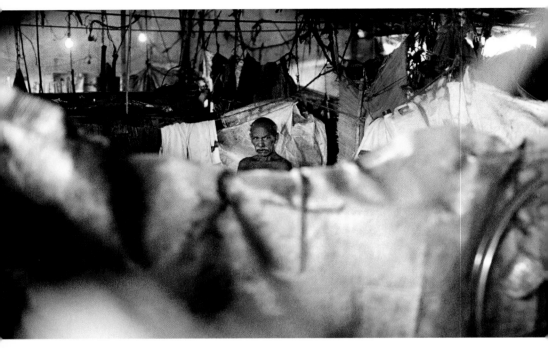

Plastic sheets offer little privacy in a camp for displaced people in Sri Lanka. A ceasefire in February 2002 allowed MSF to close some of its projects, though it still runs psychosocial programs in the country.

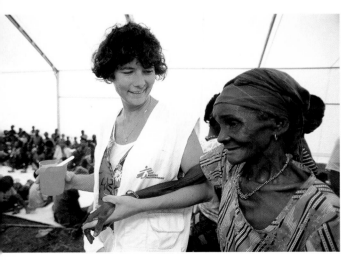

While MSF feeding centers normally treat children under five, blanket feeding programs, like this one in Liberia in 1996, also provide nutritious meals for pregnant and nursing women and the elderly.

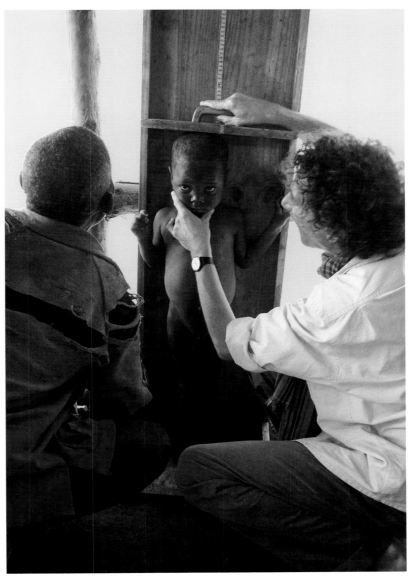

A French nurse sizes up a young boy in a refugee camp in Malawi in 1988. The child was one of hundreds of thousands who fled the civil war that plagued Mozambique from the late 1970s until 1992.

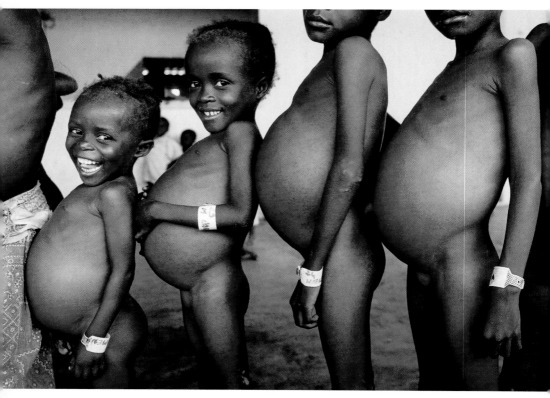

Above: With smiles that belie their suffering, children wait to be weighed at an MSF feeding center in Benguela, Angola. Their distended bellies and discolored hair are both signs of malnutrition.

Opposite: Rwandan refugees line up for water in Kibumba, Zaire, in July 1994. After Tutsi fighters halted the advance of the génocidaires, over a million Hutus fled to several camps in neighboring Zaire.

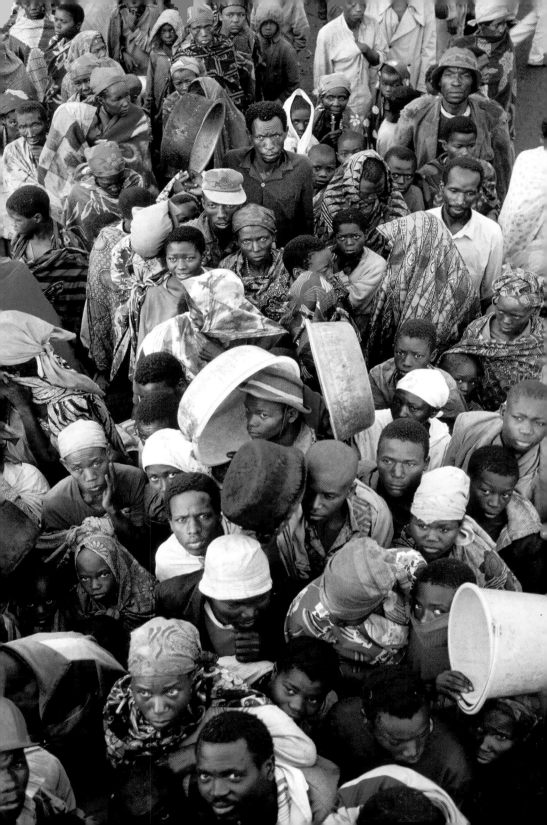

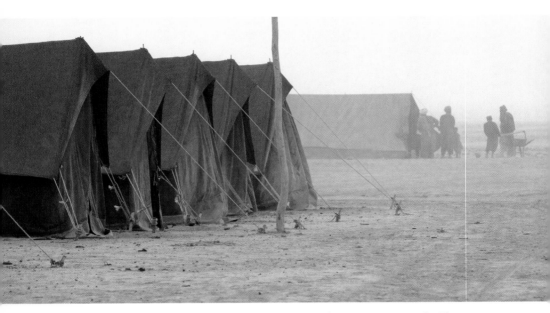

Respiratory illnesses caused by the blowing dust are common in Zhare Dasht, a camp for tens of thousands of displaced Afghans who moved there in 2002 after months in a no man's land near the Pakistani border.

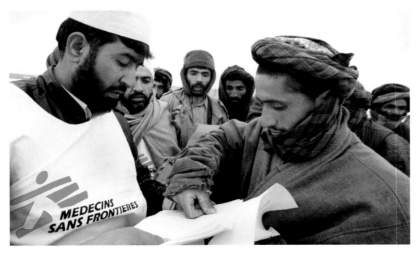

Following the ousting of the Taliban in late 2001, MSF provided health care for about 3,000 families who settled in a camp near Mazar-e-Sharif in northern Afghanistan.

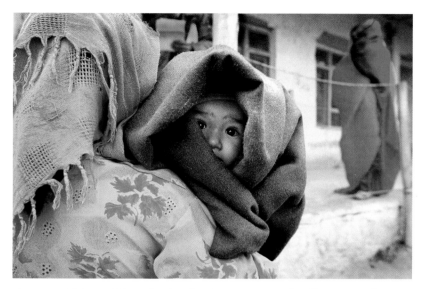

A young Afghan girl carries her brother to an MSF feeding center in Meymaneh, Afghanistan, in December 2001. Drought and war combined to make malnutrition a major problem in the region.

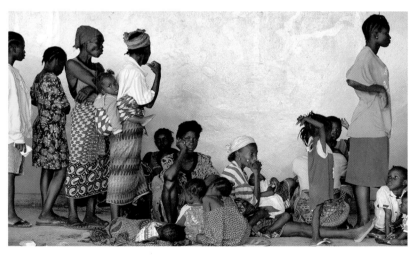

In the basement of a Monrovia sports stadium, women wait to have their children weighed and registered by MSF staff. About 15,000 displaced Liberians took refuge here when fighting erupted in the spring of 2003.

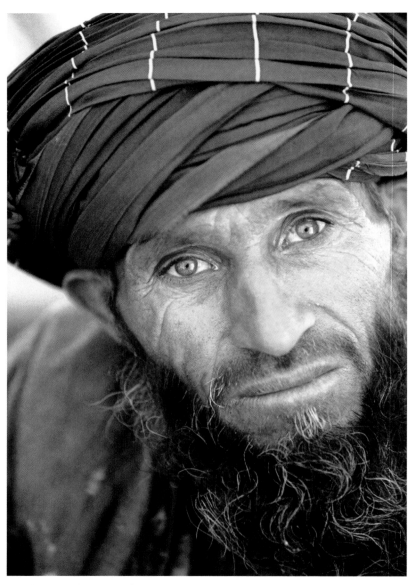

At the MSF clinic in Sar-e Pol, in northern Afghanistan in December 2001, the eyes of an elderly man reflect the resilience with which his people have endured decades of hardship.

some ways, it represents a mindset that we think is important, because the world of aid is dominated by big institutional actors – the Red Cross, UN, big NGOs – who often become integrated into governmental politics and lose sight of individual suffering. *Sans frontières* is not a cowboy mentality, but there is a rebellious element to it, which we think is an essential part of humanitarianism. You have to be willing to cross a border to attend to suffering."

The white Toyota Land Cruiser has become the standard vehicle of MSF and many other aid agencies, but sometimes projects in remote areas are inaccessible even to rugged four-wheel-drives. In the 21st century, it's easy to forget that there are still pockets of the globe that have virtually no contact with the outside world. In the summer of 2003, the Spanish section sent a doctor and nurse to do an explo in a remote area of Bamiyan province, in central Afghanistan, where they encountered people who had never seen a car before. They did part of the trip on donkeys, echoing MSF's first mission in the country two decades before, which used the same mode of four-legged transportation. One local staffer wasn't surprised by the story. He'd been part of an earlier explo mission to an area where people jumped back in fear when they heard the vehicle, calling it a monster. In South Sudan, where flooding can make roads impassable for vehicles, MSF nurses and their assistants make four- or five-day trips on bicycles to treat malaria patients. Other MSF projects have sent medical staff deep into the Congolese jungle on motorbikes or into the South American rainforest in tiny boats.

When a project involves remote terrain and a clandestine element, it can take on a cloak-and-dagger flavor. Thirteen days after returning from his first mission in Kosovo, Patrick Lemieux was back on a plane, this time headed for Congo, where MSF-Spain had just completed an explo and was setting up a new project. "They say it will be about a two-day trip to there, and after that you'll take a small plane there, and someone by the name of X will meet you, and the password is this, and they smuggle you in. It sounds much more scary in hindsight, but the idea was that we were going in on the rebel side. You can't obtain a visa – you arrive there and deal with the 'customs officers.' They want money and you tell them you don't have any."

In August 2003, Lemieux also organized an exploratory mission in Sindh province, Pakistan, which had been hit with massive flooding. MSF's plan was to reach the victims with mobile clinics – a pair of Land Cruisers that travel to remote areas to deliver medical care. As well as a doctor and a nurse, these hospitals on wheels may include a drug dispenser, a registrar to look after the paperwork and a "lady health visitor," the charming name given to women who do basic health care and outreach in rural areas. The cars are loaded with medication, intravenous fluids, health cards and stationery, foam mattresses, plastic sheeting, emergency lights, flags and stickers with the MSF logo, and jerry cans of drinking water. They set up in schools or mosques, or under a shady tree, sometimes in nameless villages that don't appear on maps and are found only with the help of a local guide. Because security wasn't an issue in Sindh province, the mobile clinics could stay overnight in the communities they visited, and the convoy could follow a more or less linear route. In dangerous regions, the cars return to a base each night and often wait until late morning before setting out again – to allow other vehicles traveling the road to set off any lurking mines.

Whether the health clinics are permanent buildings or four-wheel-drives, medical care in rural Africa has few dull moments. During a mission in Ethiopia with MSF-Belgium, physician Marie-Jo Ouimet was based in Deghabur, in the Ogaden region of the country, which is inhabited by ethnic Somalis. It's a polygamous culture, and Ouimet treated several men who had been anointed with boiling water by their jealous wives. Some of the children had serious burns from upsetting cooking pots or falling into fires. Ouimet also regularly made journeys of six hours or more to visit far-flung health posts and train local staff. On one of these overnight stays, some villagers arrived before supper with a man who had been bitten by a snake. "The health post didn't have antivenin medication, and we didn't have anything to transfuse him with," Ouimet says. "There wasn't much we could do. He wasn't very symptomatic at that point, but we kept a close eye on him at the clinic. We knew we had to take him to the referral hospital, but we had to wait until the next day, because we had strict rules never to be on the road after four o'clock for security reasons, and we had to respect that, even though we knew he might not survive. We managed to stabilize him until the morning – we were up all night adjusting the IV and giving him analgesics – and we got on the road as soon as the sun was up. Just before we left, the villagers brought the snake they thought had bitten him – I don't know if it was the actual snake, or if they just killed a snake as a kind of revenge. But after about an hour and a half, he just died in the car."

In acute emergencies, medical aid can save hundreds of lives in days or weeks. In rural health projects, however, success is far less dramatic. And while outbreaks of disease can be brought under control, doctors doing primary health care in places like Ogaden have nagging doubts about the long-term prospects of their patients. From the beginning, Ouimet wondered just how much good MSF was doing in the area. "Our project didn't make much sense, and I thought it wasn't worth taking such high risks for something that had absolutely no impact."

The risks were certainly high. There's a constant military presence in the region, as the rebel Ogaden National Liberation Front fights to annex the region to Somalia. In September 1999, when Ouimet arrived, the project had just reopened after having been shut down following direct attacks on aid agencies by the ONLF, including the kidnapping of an expat with a French NGO. "Right before the kidnapping, the rebels had intercepted an MSF car and threatened the occupants – they pointed their guns at them and told them to undress and dig their graves. Then they set the car on fire and left. I was worried, but we had a lot of rules and were very conscious about security, so I thought the risk of anything happening was pretty low. It almost became a bit of a joke. We had 'kidnapping bags' – every time we went on the road we had little backpacks with some food, mosquito repellent, matches. This was something you were supposed to be able to survive with if you were stuck in the bush without a vehicle or if you were kidnapped. It was a little bit silly, but it was part of our security guidelines."

In the new year, with elections planned, there were other security incidents in the area, and Ouimet's team talked about pulling out. Then came reports about a possible famine in the south of the region, and she was selected to fly out and do a nutritional survey. When the car dropped her off at the airport on February 7, 2000, she said goodbye to the driver, his brother, and the team's French logistician, Stéphane Courteheuse. Shortly after three in the afternoon, the staff in Deghabur tried to contact the car by radio but got no response. They dispatched a second car to investigate and discovered that Courteheuse's vehicle had been ambushed on the return drive from the airport. The driver was killed instantly by five bullets to the head, while Courteheuse was shot once in the chest during the ambush, then dragged from the car and shot again, with one of the bullets shattering his eighth dorsal vertebra. The attackers then stole his watch, his passport and his electric guitar. (The driver's brother managed to hide in the back of the car.) When the Deghabur staff arrived on the scene, the logistician was lying on the side of the road, taking water offered by some villagers.

Courteheuse was driven back to Deghabur for treatment, then to a Nairobi hospital, before eventually being evacuated home. After five months in the hospital, and now confined to a wheelchair, he returned to work in MSF's Brussels office in January 2002. Twenty-nine years old at the time of the shooting, Courteheuse was already a veteran of seven previous MSF missions, most recently in the Democratic Republic of Congo, where he had been imprisoned. He had hoped the Ethiopia mission would be a relatively easy one by comparison, but irony is another of humanitarianism's ugly realities.

In an ill-equipped health clinic with no lab, where the only diagnostic tools are your eyes and hands, it's easy to feel you've been cast adrift. "The first thing you realize is that the people who are going to save you are your staff," says nurse Leanne

Olson. "There are nursing schools everywhere in Africa. All of the nurses I worked with were trained, they had their degrees, they had studied, but we underestimate their diagnostic capacities and their ability to treat people, and we do that at great risk. They're perfectly capable of taking care of their own people – much better than I can, because they know the diseases, they know the parasites, they know what schistosomiasis looks like inside and out. They can tell me whether this is a surgical emergency or not. I learned so much by working with and understanding my national staff."

Of course, incompetent and indifferent people can hold important positions too, and, while that's true everywhere, in developing countries they can often act with impunity. In 2000, Olson was in Mile 91, a town in northern Sierra Leone, where about 40,000 displaced people had settled. MSF had set up clinics there, but the referral hospital was a couple of hours away. The man in charge of health care in the area had the habit of borrowing the MSF car whenever he pleased. "One day he took off for Freetown and I thought he would be gone for two days. Well, he was gone for *fifteen* days. I had seventeen people die from correctable surgical problems. Maybe all of them, maybe only some of them, would have lived if they had received surgery. I tried everything – I was trying to put them on buses, I was trying to find other agencies that could take them. When he came back, he didn't care."

You don't have to be a doctor or a nurse to know that countless people die in the developing world from senseless violence, or for lack of basic drugs, or because medical staff don't have the training or tools they need. But it's something quite different when those patients die on your watch. Even after eight years in the field, Olson never got used to it. "In Sierra

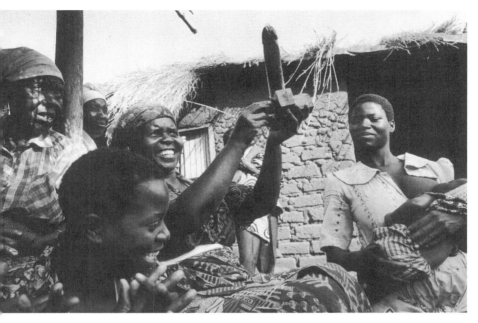

In a Malawi village where AIDS is rampant, MSF helps women learn the fine art of using a condom. While humor is usually an effective tool, expat staff often confront unfamiliar languages, customs and other cultural barriers as they deliver their health message.

Leone, I sent a mom to the hospital for surgery who had a four-month-old baby, which I didn't know, and they contacted me and said, 'The mother died. What do you want us to do with the baby?' They sent us back a four-month-old baby – and then he died of meningitis. I took a woman who desperately needed a C-section to the hospital, but the doctor was away at a meeting, so she died. And her baby died. I had to bring her husband back the next day to the village and say I was really sorry. That kind of thing is the hardest to accept in MSF."

On her first mission in Burundi, nurse Carol McCormack was part of a team that supported eight health centers in the remote Moso region, along the Tanzanian border. Each center was run by a nurse, but the rest of the national staff were just laypeople who had trained in basic procedures like hygiene and dressings. McCormack learned a little Kurundi – *Where does it hurt? Do you have a fever? Are you throwing up?* – but couldn't get over some of the cultural hurdles. "Trying to introduce condoms was one of my crusades, but it's almost crazy. They just laughed when I pulled out the wooden penis and tried to demonstrate how to use the condom.

"It was so overwhelming. We were just starting the project, and putting down on paper everything that needed to be done. Then you try to put that plan into action, and it's impossible. Every day we would go out and try to fix things, try to make the health centers better. At the beginning, people would tug on my sleeve and I would say, 'Leave me alone, go see the other nurse, I've got to organize your immunization plan.' Then one of our managers said to me, 'You know, you have to deal with the patient who's in front of you. You can't fix everybody, you can't fix the injustices and the disease, but you can help that old lady who's pointing to her son who's going blind because of vitamin A deficiency.' That really helped me get through the last few months of the mission."

Like many volunteers who have long since returned home, McCormack stills sees her patients when she closes her eyes. "Children with gunshot wounds are the ones that really stick in my head. The one I remember the most was Cesar. He was a little boy I had seen at the hospital in Ruyigi. There had been fighting in the Moso and he was shot in the elbow. He walked all the way to Ruyigi, which was probably hours and hours of walking. When he was discharged from the hospital he didn't have any place to go. He showed up at our gate, and I was going in and out that day, seeing this kid there. Finally one of the guards tapped me on the shoulder and said, 'This kid wants to talk to one of you. He doesn't have anywhere to go.' His parents had been killed in the fighting, and then his neighbors, who were his guardians, were killed too. He was twelve years old, and he didn't know where to go.

"There was a lady in town named Maggie, who ran an orphanage. So Cesar asked us if we would talk to her and see if she would let him stay with these orphans. We went to see Maggie, and of course she said he could stay. As I left, he was standing there thinking, 'Sure, I'm in this orphanage, but what do I do now? I don't know anybody.' I had to just walk away. I can deal with medical things. But a child who has nowhere to go was something I could not get my head around."

When Médecins Sans Frontières was nothing more than a good idea waiting to happen, Raymond Borel was already urging French doctors to aid victims of earthquakes, hurricanes and tsunamis. But MSF's earliest interventions in natural disasters failed – first in the Nicaraguan earthquake of 1972, and then in Honduras during Hurricane Fifi a year later – because it arrived well after rescue efforts by other agencies were already under way. Three decades later, MSF is faster and more experienced, and it is still on the ground following natural disasters. But many in the organization wonder if it should be involved in this kind of work at all.

"There's precious little that an organization like MSF can do in an earthquake," says Nabil al-Tikriti, who was part of a relief team that went to Turkey after the devastating quake of

August 17, 1999. "In an earthquake, people are dead or alive within the first three days, and you can't get much going in three days. You need to get rescue teams in there, and that's not what we do. There are other groups that are far better at it. Unless there's a public-health breakdown, there's not much of a role for us."

Of course, there are always ongoing medical needs in the wake of a disaster like the Turkey earthquake, which killed more than 16,000 people and left some 600,000 homeless. MSF had four teams in the hardest-hit cities within a week, along with 30 tons of medical supplies, tents and other shelters. The teams included specialists in treating kidney failure, a common and potentially fatal ailment in people who have survived "crush syndrome" – internal injuries from collapsed buildings. MSF also installed huge bladders to supply some 15,000 people with fresh water. So even if its staff isn't pulling victims from the rubble, MSF can play a useful role in disaster relief. But with limited resources, the question is whether funds and volunteers might be better deployed elsewhere. As al-Tikriti points out, even an organization that can afford to snub institutional donors can still be influenced by the well-meaning citizen who asks that her check go to help the people she's seen on the news.

"Private donors are very trusting of MSF to be stewards of their funds," al-Tikriti says, "and they should be, because MSF has a good record, and I would vouch for that." While donors can earmark their money for certain crises, he says, most do not, except when something dramatic like a natural disaster dominates the news for several days. When that happens, ad hoc donations can dramatically exceed what is needed for a relatively short-term relief effort.

The South Asian tsunami in December 2004 was hardly a short-term crisis, but MSF knew quickly that bringing medical aid to the survivors would not require the huge sums that immediately poured in from donors. Within a week of the disaster, MSF posted a notice on its website asking the public not to direct money to tsunami relief because they had sufficient funds already. When it became clear that there would be no mass outbreak of cholera or other water-borne disease, MSF recognized that its post-tsunami role would be relatively limited. They chose to focus on Aceh, Indonesia, where medical needs were most acute, and to leave the long-term rebuilding to other organizations better equipped to the task.

Nonetheless, by the end of March 2005, donors around the world had sent MSF more than €105 million (about $130 million) for tsunami victims, while the budgeters believed only a quarter of that total would be needed to extend its efforts to the end of the year. This left the organization with a dilemma: was it ethical to spend these excess millions on another crisis? MSF decided the right move was to contact the donors and ask them for permission to direct their contribution to underfunded projects in Africa. Overwhelmingly, the donors said yes – more than half the money has since been redistributed, and less than 1 percent was refunded.

While MSF has no intention of getting involved in reconstruction after natural disasters, it has found an ongoing role in psychosocial programs – its post-tsunami projects, for example, all have a mental-health components that have continued past the emergency phase. Long after victims are buried and destroyed homes are rebuilt, the psychological wounds of survivors linger. Following an earthquake, up to 60 percent of adults and 95 percent of children may suffer from post-traumatic stress disorder, so MSF sends psychologists to counsel victims and, more often, train local counselors to deal with the aftermath. Still a relatively new part of MSF's field-work, mental-health programs have had limited success. Some have stretched the mandate of a medical organization, involving community artists, storytellers, even gardeners and expat drama therapists. Indeed, there's some controversy as to whether mental-health programs should be part of emergency relief at all, or, instead, a low priority that can be tackled after more acute medical needs have been met. Few would deny, however, that an effective mental-health program will not only help people rebuild their lives in the long term but also reduce the strain on the medical system in the weeks and months after an emergency.

Adrienne Carter, a psychologist who has worked with MSF in Kosovo, Sri Lanka and Kashmir, says that outpatient doctors in crisis zones often deal with patients for only a few minutes before hastily prescribing drugs. "Valium is given like candy," she says, as people show up with headaches, stomach pains, sleep problems and other psychosomatic symptoms. One MSF doctor working with long-time refugees says that up to 40 percent of the ailments he saw at his outpatient clinic had a psychological basis.

For people uprooted by war, forced to live on the run or in crowded camps, psychological problems go far beyond aches and pains. "Sri Lanka was one of the worst situations we had seen," Carter says. She was in the country in 2002, working with minority Tamils, who are still recovering from two decades of war with the Sinhalese-dominated government. The conflict claimed some 64,000 lives and displaced hundreds of thousands of people. Many Tamils had been kidnapped, detained and beaten, had faced starvation or seen family members burned alive inside their homes. In one MSF survey of displaced people in the town of Vavuniya, 88 percent said they felt constantly unsafe.

In the Tamil camps, Carter saw the consequences of this insecurity. "It was a complete breakdown of moral values. Everything that could happen did happen. Normally in Tamil communities, families are very strong and very supportive of each other, but the breakdowns among the internally displaced were just brutal. A lot of them turned to a home-brewed liquor that was widely used in the camps, and many became addicted, which meant that even if they were able to find jobs, they couldn't work, so families broke apart with amazing ease. Fathers just deserted their families and shacked up with another family, so children had absolutely no stability. Food wasn't coming regularly, so everything was extremely unstable, and these people had lived like that for the past ten to fifteen years. And their environment was so horrible. Tiny, tiny places that were separated from the next family by plastic sheets, so there was no privacy at all.

"There was a school in the camps, but often kids did not attend, and there wasn't enough supervision from the parents or anyone else. These were some of the things that our workers were trying to help. One of the huge issues was that people had no problem-solving ability whatsoever – if an issue came up, they would turn to suicide before trying to solve it. Suicides were committed or threatened for what we might think of as very mild issues like, 'I had a fight with my aunt, so I'm going to kill myself.'"

Perhaps no type of project requires more cultural sensitivity than one that addresses mental health, and MSFers admit they've made many mistakes, though they've also pioneered some successful techniques. Carter was surprised when a phone-in show MSF arranged on a local radio station in Kosovo was so popular – despite having to use an on-air translator – that it was invited back for weeks. The anonymity of the radio allowed people to ask freely about sexual dysfunction, a common symptom of stress. As a bonus, the psychologists' answers were heard by far more people than MSF could hope to counsel in person.

In Kashmir, the disputed Muslim area between India and Pakistan, Carter remembers there was an outcry when her team wanted to train male and female sexual-abuse counselors together. Eventually they agreed to divide the group by gender, though Carter ended up being the only woman in a room of 15 or 20 men. As is usual in crisis areas, those being trained were almost all victims themselves. "You couldn't even look them in the face – I did it without any eye contact. There was complete quiet in the room. And then one man started very haltingly to speak about his own torture and abuse. Then another, and another. It was an incredibly heavy two hours, as they chose to share their experiences. This would never have happened if there were women there."

Even when MSF psychologists have the opportunity to counsel patients directly, they can't always get the same gratification as a surgeon who removes a bullet or cures a baby with malaria. There are no quick fixes for traumatized people. "In this work, you grow so close to the people that you can't just leave them, arrive back home, and let them out of your heart," says Carter. "Each time I vow that I'm not going to become attached, I'm just going to do my job. It never works."

7 | How the Other Half Dies

James Orbinski traveled a long and painful road on his way to the Oslo City Hall podium on December 10, 1999. The Canadian doctor received his medical degree at McMaster University in Hamilton, Ontario, in 1990, and less than three years later found himself in Somalia with Médecins Sans Frontières during the famine, civil war and botched US intervention. When he returned home, he knew things had changed in him forever. As he gave advice to a patient in his small-town practice, a mother having difficulty breastfeeding, she mentioned that his mind seemed to be elsewhere. Orbinski admitted she was right, and when she left his office he sat silently for 20 minutes and realized he couldn't do this kind of medicine anymore. He closed his office and went back into the field with MSF, first to Afghanistan and later to Rwanda, arriving a month after the genocide had begun. During one of those terrible days in 1994, Orbinski tried to negotiate with a Hutu commander whose killing squad had surrounded a building filled with Tutsi children. "There was a long pause," he later told a journalist. "He looked at me and said, 'These are insects and they will be crushed like insects.'" When the doctor returned the next day, a blue tarp covered the bodies of the children who had been hacked to death.

Orbinski suffered from post-traumatic stress disorder for a year and a half after the genocide – he would see that tarp in his mind over and over, the memory triggered by passing blue cars as he drove along the highway. But whatever ghosts still haunted him in 1996, he was back in Africa, working among the Rwandan refugees who had fled to Zaire. In 1998 he became the international president of MSF, the first non-European to hold the position. Orbinski is a medical researcher, with a specialty in pediatric HIV, but, like Rony Brauman and other charismatic former leaders of MSF, he's also a philosopher with a keen understanding of politics (and a master's degree in international relations). During his three-year tenure as international president, he met with some of the organization's other big thinkers – including Brauman, Austen Davis, and Jean-Marie Kindermans – to try to draft a mission statement that would illuminate the MSF charter in a way that all the national sections could agree on. At one point, they had at least a dozen sections on side, but no document had been approved. Just then, on October 15, 1999, the news arrived that Médecins Sans Frontières had been awarded the Nobel Peace Prize "in recognition of the organization's pioneering humanitarian work on several continents." MSF decided to use this opportunity to lay out its mission in a much more public forum – the Nobel acceptance lecture, delivered by Orbinski in Norway that December.

In a provocative opening, Orbinski set aside diplomatic

niceties and immediately called for the Russian government "to stop the bombing of defenseless civilians in Chechnya." He outlined the humanitarian impulses that have guided the organization over three decades. Then he went on to announce what would become MSF's next crusade. "More than ninety percent of all death and suffering from infectious diseases occurs in the developing world," Orbinski said, and tropical illnesses are killing people because "life-saving essential medicines are either too expensive, or not available because they are not seen as financially viable, or because there is virtually no new research and development" into new treatments. "This market failure," he declared, "is our next challenge."

And so it was. Along with the Nobel gold medal and diploma, MSF picked up a check for 7.9 million Swedish crowns, equivalent to just over a million US dollars. It wasn't the largest donation MSF has ever received, but it packed more symbolic punch than any other. MSF decided to use the money to kick-start the Campaign for Access to Essential Medicines.

The term "essential medicines" isn't just rhetoric. It refers to a list drawn up by the World Health Organization and includes more than three hundred drugs – for everything from HIV to gout – that are considered the minimum needed to set up a basic health-care system. The Access campaign, however, focuses on the developing world's deadliest diseases, each of which has a unique set of barriers to treatment. There's leishmaniasis, a parasitical disease in Asia and Africa, currently treated with a 60-year-old drug that is unaffordable for most patients. Sleeping sickness, or human African trypanosomiasis, is carried by the tsetse fly in sub-Saharan Africa and is also treated with a decades-old drug that faces growing resistance – it's so toxic that it burns when injected, and it fatally poisons up to a tenth of those who receive it. Tuberculosis kills 2 million people a year and is increasingly drug resistant because most patients do not follow the entire nine-month treatment regimen. As for meningitis, an effective vaccine is available, but too few doses are being manufactured and too little money is pledged to administer them.

Pharmaceutical companies devote little or no research to new treatments for these and other tropical diseases because the promise of profit is negligible compared with drugs for erectile dysfunction, hair loss, obesity and wrinkles. To change this trend, MSF helped found the Drugs for Neglected Diseases Initiative, which coordinates new research and development into ailments that have been ignored by the profit-driven drug industry. This initiative has been the most internally controversial part of the Access campaign, with some arguing that MSF should not be involved in long-term lobbying or R&D. In 2002, after an otherwise unanimous vote in the International Council, MSF-Holland refused to help fund DNDi, as it is called. The dispute dragged on for more than a year before the Dutch reluctantly gave in. In the opinion of many, it reignited the strife between sections that MSF had worked so hard to overcome.

In other ways, however, the campaign's grand scope has brought together MSFers of many backgrounds – not only the doctors and nurses in the field, but also a determined team of lawyers, pharmacists and lobbyists. Nowhere is this more true than in the fight to deliver treatment for malaria, the infectious disease that has probably killed more human beings than any other in history, and AIDS, the scourge that's poised to take over that dubious honor.

Unlike leishmaniasis and sleeping sickness, malaria is well known to everyone in the West, though today it's largely thought of as a historical curiosity like smallpox or the Black Death. Yet it was endemic in many developed countries only a few decades ago – Holland did not eradicate it until after World War II. Today, while industrialized countries pour money into public-health bugaboos like avian influenza, West Nile virus and severe acute respiratory syndrome, malaria quietly kills up to 2 million people every year, mostly children, and 90 percent of them in Africa. To give some perspective: SARS caused fewer than eight hundred deaths worldwide in 2003, while malaria kills about the same number every six hours. For those who need to put monetary figures on this body count, the World Health Organization estimates the annual economic cost of malaria in Africa is $12 billion.

At the root of this devastation are a single-celled organism with an insatiable lust for hemoglobin and a tiny insect with a taste for human blood. Although malaria has been known for centuries, its cause was a mystery until 1880, when French doctor Charles-Louis-Alphonse Laveran used a primitive microscope to examine a malarial blood sample and became the first person to observe the *Plasmodium* parasite that causes the disease. Seventeen years later, British physician Ronald Ross, working in India, proved that this parasite is transmitted to humans by mosquitoes, a discovery that earned him a Nobel Prize in 1902. About 30 species of mosquito – all in the genus *Anopheles* – are significant carriers, and when females bite humans they deposit *Plasmodium* sporozoites into the bloodstream. These spores convene in the liver, where they marshal themselves for two to four weeks before launching an all-out assault on the red blood cells. Once inside the red cells, the parasites feed voraciously on hemoglobin, the substance that carries oxygen around the body. They reproduce quickly and eventually burst through the cell membrane, releasing their offspring to infect other red blood cells.

Four species of *Plasmodium* cause malaria in humans, although one – *P. falciparum* – is far more deadly than the others. In addition to fever, symptoms of the disease include chills, muscle aches, headaches, abdominal pain, vomiting, diarrhea and general malaise, though they vary from mild discomfort to sheer misery. Severe malaria can cause jaundice, kidney failure or abnormal bleeding, and the *falciparum* parasite can enter the brain's bloodstream – a condition called cerebral malaria – leading to delirium, convulsions, coma and potentially death. In children, *falciparum* malaria can also kill by causing severe anemia. Adults in endemic areas who have survived repeated infections eventually build up some immunity and usually endure subsequent bouts with only minor symptoms. (Travelers – including MSF expats – who visit endemic areas have none of this immunity and can become severely ill if they fail to take precautions, such as sleeping under a bed net, using insect repellent and taking malaria prophylaxis.) The exception is pregnant women, who lose their immunity and can become dangerously anemic if they contract malaria. Moreover, the parasites converge on the placenta – so much so that they may barely register elsewhere in the body – and retard the growth of the fetus. When these babies are born, they are often too small to survive.

Even in areas where malaria is endemic, it can be extremely difficult to diagnose in underequipped health centers. Ideally, a lab technician should examine the blood for parasites under a microscope; where this is impossible, MSF uses a rapid blood test – similar in principle to a home pregnancy test – that takes only 15 minutes. Done rigorously, both methods are around 90 percent accurate, but lack of training and time lessen that reliability. For doctors who rely only on observing symptoms, malaria is notoriously hard to identify, since many unrelated conditions cause fever, chills and aches. While the diagnosis in young children is often accurate, MSF doctors have worked in areas where 80 percent of adults and kids over five who are thought to have malaria are actually suffering from something else. This misdiagnosis not only leads to wasted medicines and more potential for the drugs to encounter resistance, but also means those patients are enduring some other illness – such as hepatitis, meningitis, pneumonia or typhoid – that's going untreated. Some end up back in the hospital days or weeks later, while others die at home.

Malaria occupies an important place in pharmacological history. As far back as the 1630s – when doctors still thought illness was caused by an imbalance of blood, bile and phlegm – Jesuit missionaries in Peru discovered that the bark of the cinchona tree, when ground into powder, could be used to cure malarial fever. It was the first time that a chemical compound – later identified as quinine – was successfully used to treat an infectious disease. Almost four centuries later, quinine is still an effective treatment in Africa, but it can have truly unpleasant side effects, including nausea and tinnitus (ringing in the ears), and it is toxic in large doses. Taken orally, quinine is unpalatably bitter, and if delivered intravenously it requires three daily injections. Either way, treatment takes a full week, which can strain the resources of a crowded health center.

In the first half of the 20th century, two new discoveries promised to wipe out malaria for good – chloroquine, a drug first developed in 1934, and the insecticide DDT, introduced in the 1940s. A massive international effort to spray mosquito breeding grounds in the 1950s and 1960s helped eradicate the disease from parts of Europe and Asia, and even in Africa malaria rates declined into the 1980s. By then, however, the *falciparum* parasite had developed a resistance to chloroquine in many areas. In the 1990s, doctors were encouraged by sulfadoxine-pyrimethamine (SP), but again the adaptable parasite quickly developed a resistance to this treatment, too. MSF now considers chloroquine and SP "virtually useless" in much of sub-Saharan Africa. One or the other, however, is still the first-line treatment in most of these countries.

In October 2002, MSF announced its intention to replace these drugs in all its malaria projects with a two-drug cocktail called artemisinin-based combination therapy, or ACT. Artemisinin, like quinine, is extracted from a plant whose medicinal qualities have been tapped for centuries – an aromatic herb, *Artemisia annua*, known in its native China as *qinghaosu* and in the West as sweet Annie, or sweet wormwood. The herb yields a substance that is not only swift and effective in treating malaria – it kills parasites 10 times faster than quinine – but has virtually no side effects. Used alone, artemisinin-based drugs such as artesunate and artemether relieve symptoms in a day or two, though it takes about a week to clear the body of parasites. However, when they are combined with another antimalarial drug – such as amodiaquine, lumefantrine, mefloquine or even SP if there is no resistance – treatment can be shortened to three days, a regimen people are much more likely to complete. More important, the one-two punch of ACT radically reduces the likelihood that *P. falciparum* will fight back. The parasite already needs to undergo several mutations to defeat a single drug, so the chances of developing a resistance to two drugs simultaneously are remote. In the decade or so that MSF has used artemisinin combinations – admittedly on a small scale, mainly in Southeast Asia, and in a few feeding centers and refugee camps in Africa – they have shown no sign of losing their potency.

MSF failed to meet its target date of bringing ACT into widespread use in Africa by the end of 2003, though the organization estimates that it treated 100,000 patients with the therapy that year. It has faced a number of challenges, beginning with what MSF sees as the reluctance of public-health decision makers to get behind the new drug. The general trend in malaria control is toward prevention – spraying during epidemics and distributing insecticide-treated bed nets – rather than treatment. The Global Fund to Fight AIDS, Tuberculosis and Malaria has pledged $30 million over five years to purchase artemisinin-based drugs, and Roll Back Malaria – a WHO-founded joint venture – has called them "the way forward for treating malaria." But all these initiatives are moving far too slowly for MSF. In November 2003, the organization assembled an international team of malaria experts and drafted a letter to Roll Back Malaria, arguing that its new four-year plan was "a backward step in malarial control" that would "reverse more than five years of consultation and expert opinion." As for other NGOs that are still using the older drugs, UK physician Christa Hook, one of the architects of MSF's malaria strategy, puts their resistance down to financial dependence on Western governments, and an inclination "not to pioneer."

"The other main problem," says Hook, "is that in some countries there's a very strong bureaucracy, a very strong ministry of health that is not allowing us to use ACT. Within such

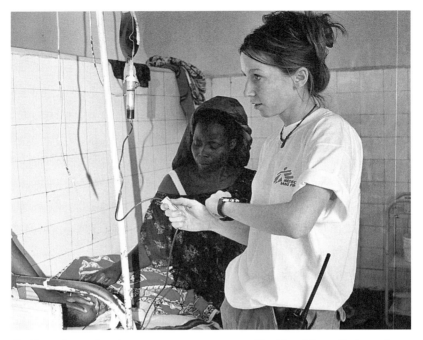

In Man, Ivory Coast, an MSF nurse oversees the blood transfusion of a baby with cerebral malaria while the mother looks on. Eradicated in the West, malaria kills up to two million people a year in the developing world, largely because the parasite is increasingly resistant to the drugs used to treat it.

countries, we sometimes have totally independent facilities – for example, we might run a mobile clinic, or a therapeutic feeding center, which is not ministry of health at all – where we can introduce ACT, despite the country not changing its policy. We've used it in refugee camps because, again, they're separate – they're run entirely by NGOs, or UNHCR."

MSF has grown accustomed to ruffling the feathers of UN agencies and other aid organizations, but its zeal for artemisinin has even rankled health ministries in some of the countries where it works. In Ethiopia, where a malaria epidemic threatened 15 million people in 2003, MSF lobbied hard for the immediate introduction of artemisinin combinations, only to find opposition from UNICEF, the local WHO official and the Ethiopian authorities. The health ministry argued that it was inappropriate and unethical to introduce a treatment in the middle of an epidemic and preferred to wait for the results of its own studies before introducing ACT. On December 23, health minister Kebede Tadesse attacked MSF in a bombastic press release:

[MSF's] track record is exemplary and we are very grateful to the many devoted volunteers for their unreserved contributions ... However, for reasons not well known to us, and based on their totally unscientific and unverifiable observations of the present malaria situation in a few localities, [they] have embarked on a concerted campaign of misinformation and peddling of new and uncalled for drugs and treatment regimes. We have tried to reason out with them repeatedly, but they have become unamenable to ration [sic] and are progressively resorting to dictatorial mechanisms to have their views and ways of doing things accepted. We would like to point out that any health authority of a sovereign and democratic country, however poor and short of essential resources it may be, is duty-bound to strictly follow the rules and regulations set by its government ... It is unbecoming of MSF to try to disrupt such norms and good standards of ethical practice, so as to fit with their newly acquired whims and erroneous expectations ...
It is obvious that they are unfairly taking advantage of their access to reputable journalists and media and the

unlimited time and resources at their disposal, which we are unfortunately less endowed with. We would like to take this opportunity to publicly appeal to MSF leadership, once again, to come to their senses, and restrain from unnecessarily diverting us from our primary and urgent task of attending to the sick and alleviating their sufferings. It pains us to see a once exemplary organization being led by charlatans masquerading as the sole agents of medical and scientific knowledge and wasting valuable time in activities far beyond their commendable humanitarian mandate, which by the way, is still in high demand.

Hardly anyone now questions the effectiveness of ACT, and Hook rejects the argument that it's untested – some combinations have been used since the 1980s and their safety has been well documented. The one exception is in treating women in the first trimester of pregnancy; for them, only quinine is safe and effective. What, then, is behind the objections to the new treatment? The main issue is price. A full course of ACT costs at least 60 cents per child and between $1.00 and $2.50 per adult, compared with 10 cents to treat an adult with chloroquine or SP. The current supply of artemisinin-based drugs is also limited – there is certainly not enough to treat 300 million new cases a year – and the drugs have a relatively brief shelf life of three or four years. Of course, it's a catch-22 situation – production will increase and prices will drop only when big donors commit to buying large quantities.

Aside from cost, even health ministries that acknowledge the benefits of ACT want to move cautiously to determine the best drug pairing and to gain experience in administering the new treatment. Ideally, the two medications would be put together in a "fixed dose combination," a single pill to be taken once a day. As of 2004, however, just two companies were manufacturing such a pill. The next best option is combining two individual pills in a blister pack, which makes it clear they need to be taken together. Artemisinin-based drugs can also be given by daily intravenous or intramuscular injections.

Finally, a few governments worry that if they treat some patients with ACT now, they'll set a precedent they won't be able to sustain. "It's a fair concern," says Hook, but she wonders why UNICEF won't pledge itself to that goal. "Nobody expects countries to pay for all their vaccines – UNICEF pays for the lot. So why do they make a difference between vaccine-preventable disease and diseases which kill a damn sight more children, like malaria?" Hook was encouraged that UNICEF joined MSF in co-sponsoring a symposium on ACT in April 2004. "Hopefully, we are entering a new phase of cooperation, with clarity about the need to change to effective drugs. It will certainly make a big difference if UNICEF speaks out."

For Christa Hook, the debate comes down to a fundamental humanitarian idea. "If you treat and cure one person with malaria, then you've done good. And if you introduce the treatment into a refugee camp, or a crisis where malaria is even worse than it normally would be, I can't see people saying, 'We can't do it next year, so we won't do it this year.' That's nonsense. I think it's totally wrong to say to someone, 'I'm sorry, I've got the means to save you, but I don't want to think that next year maybe I couldn't.' We try to make sure that treatment will be available next year, but we can't guarantee it. And it's not MSF's job to guarantee it, it's the country's job. Sometimes we get field people from very developmental backgrounds who don't want to do anything unless they can see what's going to happen in ten years' time. Ten years' time can take care of itself – there might be a vaccine by then. Let's save the people who are dying this year."

There's a story that's made the rounds in MSF about a patient in Kenya, a teacher suffering from AIDS-related meningitis. His drug regimen, which offered no hope of a cure, cost about $20 a day, and after exhausting his savings in a few weeks, the man began to sell his furniture and possessions. When that money ran out too, he planned to sell his house. An MSF physician eventually talked him out of that decision, which would have left the man's family with nothing, and instead helped the teacher plan for his inevitable death. The doctor wondered why, instead of being able to prolong his patient's life with affordable medicines, he was reduced to making funeral arrangements. That feeling of helplessness goes some way in explaining why AIDS has become the highest-profile disease in MSF's Access campaign.

Malaria and AIDS differ not only in their pathology and the way they're transmitted but in hugely important cultural ways. With proper treatment, malaria can be quickly and completely cured; people infected with HIV, in contrast, need daily medication for the rest of their lives. Malaria carries no stigma and presents far fewer societal hurdles for doctors delivering treatment. Perhaps most important, at least when it comes to fighting for access to medicines, HIV infects more than a million

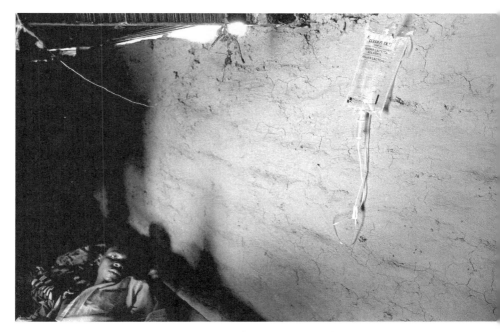

An HIV-positive patient in Zambia waits for a house call from an MSF doctor. AIDS is one of the most important target diseases in the Access to Essential Medicines campaign, which has helped to dramatically lower the price of antiretroviral drugs for people with HIV.

and a half people in North America and Europe. That means there is a vocal, well-funded, and well-organized group of activists in the West who are willing to be advocates for HIV-infected people in the developing world. And that pressure seems to be having an impact.

The United Nations estimates that more than 40 million people in poor countries are living with the virus and, of the 6 million patients who require immediate antiretroviral (ARV) treatment, only about 8 percent are getting it. (The UN's goal – with the slogan "3 by 5" – is to see that 3 million are receiving the drugs by 2005.) Aid agencies have been almost paralyzed by these overwhelming needs, and many within MSF feel the organization was too slow to get involved in HIV treatment. The Belgian office established a free and anonymous AIDS clinic in Brussels in 1988, when much of the world was still in denial about the global scope of disease, but by 2001 the organization as a whole was treating just six hundred AIDS patients in eight projects worldwide. Before 2003, the Belgians were active only in South Africa and Thailand. MSF-France treated its first patient with ARV triple therapy (a combination of three drugs that prevent the virus from replicating) in late 2000 in Thailand, while MSF-Holland showed "no real commitment to HIV until November 2002," admits Richard Bedell, who cites a number of reasons for these delays. To begin with, HIV programs, like those targeting malaria, were focused on prevention until 1996, when triple therapy emerged to make treatment possible. The drugs can now cut mortality rates by more than 80 percent. Although medical humanitarian organizations recognize that disease prevention is important, they don't always see a role there for themselves – certainly it has never been at the core of MSF's work. "But it just became more and more obvious that we couldn't turn away from this," Bedell says. "It was too important, too compelling. There's a powerful humanitarian argument for AIDS treatment. We don't know that it will change the epidemiology, but by demonstrating that people with HIV are worthy of being cared for, you humanize the whole disease, you change the attitude toward it." Once the commitment was there, MSF's programs grew rapidly, with the goal of bringing ARV therapy to 25,000 patients in 25 countries by the end of 2004.

MSF decision makers continue to feel overwhelmed by the scope of the AIDS crisis and wonder how a single NGO with

3,000 volunteers can really have an impact. "This is a huge problem that requires society-altering changes," says Bedell. "We're not the WHO, we can't do all of that. Meanwhile, the whole range of other humanitarian needs hasn't disappeared, of course." Moreover, before an organization can begin treating people for HIV, many other systems have to be in place – including the means for testing and counseling people confidentially, and an effective program for treating tuberculosis, the leading cause of death in HIV-infected people. Of the 6,000 patients receiving ARVs in MSF-France projects in 2004, up to two-thirds had TB. Most important of all, you need affordable drugs, and before 2002 there simply were none. The price of triple therapy was at least $10,000 per person every year. "We would have a hard time justifying the use of ten thousand dollars a year on a very small number of patients," Bedell says, "unless we thought it was part of a strategy to move toward something cheaper."

It *was* part of a strategy – one that goes way beyond MSF, of course, and includes Oxfam, Health Action International and innumerable other activists. Together, they succeeded in driving down the price of ARVs in 2002, and less than two years later generic versions could be bought in some countries for as little as $200 annually per patient. The work has been grueling – it's taken humanitarians into the byzantine world of patent law and international trade summits – and it's far from over. But even MSF admits the drop in prices happened more quickly than even their most optimistic forecasts.

At the center of the issue are the patents that countries grant to pharmaceutical companies, giving them a monopoly and the right to charge prices that exponentially exceed their production costs. Between 1986 and 1994 – a period that saw AIDS grow into a global pandemic – the World Trade Organization drew up the Agreement on Trade-Related Aspects of Intellectual Property Rights, or TRIPS. National governments still have widely different laws covering copyright, patents and other intellectual property, but TRIPS sets minimum guidelines that all member countries eventually have to follow, such as making sure that patented products, including medicines, are protected from competition for at least 20 years.

However, TRIPS allows governments, at least ostensibly, to make certain exceptions. For example, governments may issue "compulsory licenses" that permit local manufacturers to produce and sell cheaper generic versions of a patented drug during a public health crisis. A similar provision allows "parallel importing," or the right to purchase generic drugs from another country without the permission of the patent holder. These generic drugs – often manufactured in India or China – can be bought for a fraction of the cost that patent holders charge because their manufacturers don't have a monopoly and don't have to recoup money invested in research or clinical trials. The drugs are of comparable quality, and they must be approved by the same national authorities that approve the patented variety. They offer another benefit as well. In triple therapy for HIV, for example, the three drugs may be patented by three different companies with no interest in combining them. A generic firm, however, can put them into a single pill and make it much easier for patients to stay on their regimen. The Indian generic manufacturer Cipla offers a popular fixed-dose combination called Triomune.

The flexibility in the TRIPS agreement was supposed to balance two legitimate interests – the right of a company to benefit from its investment in R&D, and the right of people to

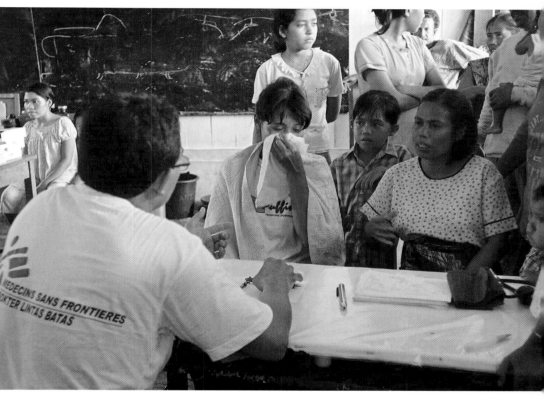

A 31-year-old woman in Aceh, Indonesia, describes how she lost her mother and three children in the tsunami of December 2004. MSF focused its tsunami relief, including mental health programs, in this hard-hit area.

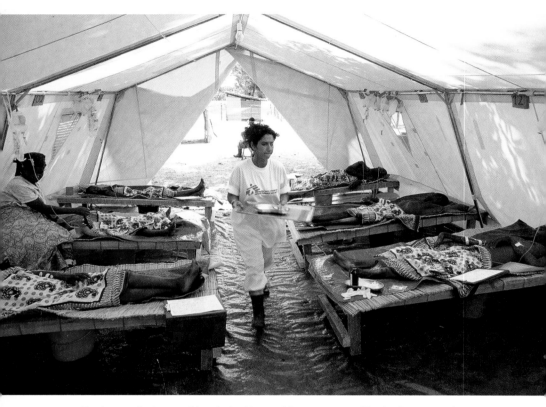

During a cholera epidemic in Mozambique, MSF staff rehydrates patients with IV drips that need to be replenished every half hour. To deal with the prodigious diarrhea, the beds have a hole in the center and a bucket underneath.

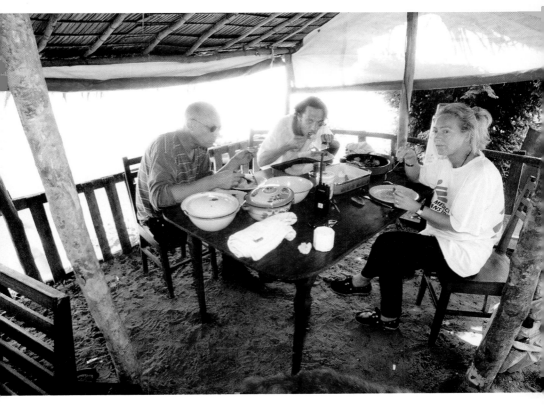

MSF volunteers enjoy an outdoor lunch in Brazzaville, Congo. Because expats arrive with widely different backgrounds, team dynamics are an unpredictable but crucially important factor in the success of a project.

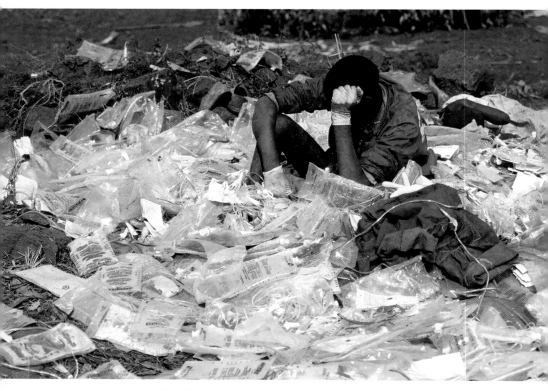

An MSF national staff member gives in to despair among the detritus of a refugee camp in Munigi, Zaire, in July 1994. Even the most seasoned aid workers were traumatized during and after the Rwandan genocide.

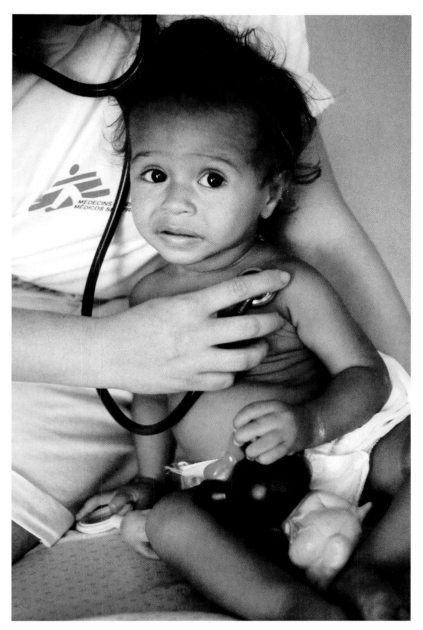

A doctor examines a baby in Vigário Giral, a slum in Rio de Janeiro. In addition to its work in conflict zones and remote areas, MSF also delivers care to the urban poor in South America, Asia, even Europe.

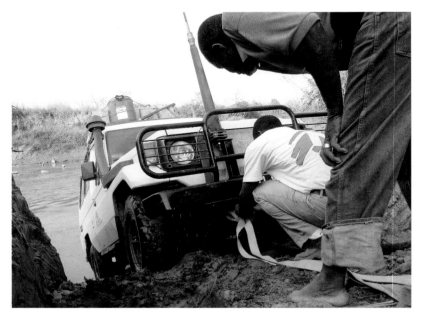

After getting stuck in the mud near Malanje, Angola, a driver attaches a strap to a Land Cruiser and attempts to pull it free. Teams traveling the roads may also have to contend with mines and ambushes.

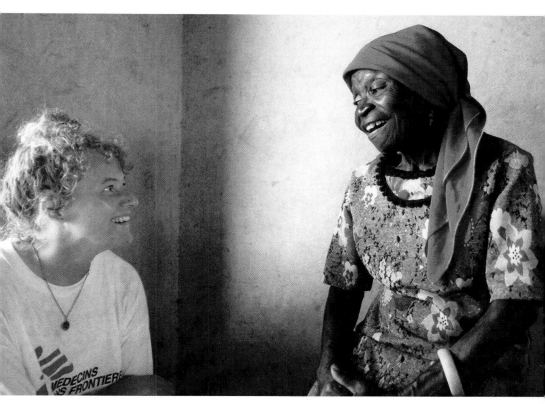

An elderly Liberian nurse chats with an MSF volunteer in a hospital in Tubmanburg. Expats rely heavily on the experience of national staff when treating local illnesses.

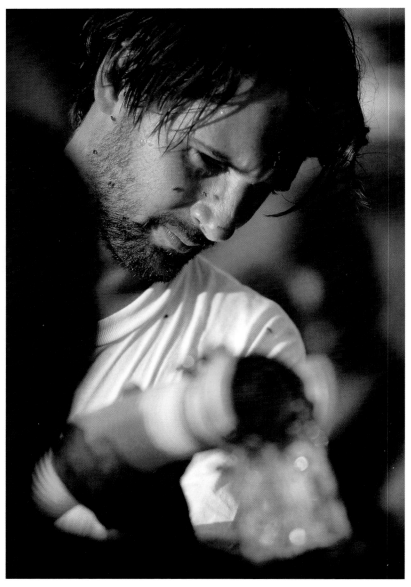

A reliable supply of fresh water is essential for running therapeutic feeding centers, which focus on children under five. During Operation Lifeline Sudan, MSF set up TFCs in many parts of the country, including this one in Ajiep.

purchase life-saving medicines at an affordable price. The problem is that rich countries have a greater stake in the former, while poorer nations gain from the latter, setting the stage for an unfair fight. And the TRIPS provisions are vague, leaving African countries to wonder how liberally they can interpret them without facing reprisals from wealthy countries with powerful pharmaceutical lobbies. It didn't take long to find out. When South Africa passed a law in 1997 that allowed the import of generic drugs to treat AIDS, it was immediately challenged by 39 drug companies. After four years of intense pressure from AIDS patients and international organizations – including MSF, whose "Drop the Case" petition garnered 293,000 signatures – the companies backed down in the face of overwhelmingly bad PR. In the meantime, hundreds of thousands of South Africans succumbed to AIDS.

In the wake of that dispute, African nations asked that the trade agreement be clarified at the WTO's ministerial conference in Doha, Qatar, in November 2001. In the months leading up to that summit, antiretrovirals for developing countries were the focus of the battle for access to affordable generic medicines. Then something happened to bring the issue home for North Americans.

In October, just weeks after the terrorist attacks on New York and Washington, five people died in the United States after opening letters laced with anthrax spores. In response, millions of North Americans clamored for ciprofloxacin, an antibiotic that can be used for anthrax prophylaxis. In both the United States and Canada, this drug was patented by Bayer Corporation and sold under the name Cipro, to the tune of over a billion dollars a year. With the increased demand during the anthrax scare, Bayer charged pharmacies a wholesale price of \$4.67 per 500-milligram tablet; a one-month supply, then, would cost the average American over \$700. Meanwhile, in India, where ciprofloxacin is not patented, Bayer was selling it in a competitive market for about \$17 a month – and still making a profit.

When the US Department of Health and Human Services asked Bayer to provide 100 million doses for its emergency stockpiles, the company offered them at \$1.83 apiece – a considerable discount, but still far more than the government was willing to pay. Health and Human Services reportedly discussed invoking the TRIPS provisions and a little-used US law to get around Bayer's patent, since generic manufacturers were offering them ciprofloxacin for as little as 40 cents a pill. Health Canada, which also has strict limits on compulsory licensing, actually placed an order with a generic manufacturer, though it later canceled the deal after Bayer threatened to sue. In the end, neither government violated the patent – it's not even clear that the United States seriously considered doing so, knowing that its double standard would be exploited in the upcoming Doha conference. In any case, Bayer was compelled to reduce its price radically to 95 cents a dose, and both countries got a taste of what it was like to have a potentially life-saving drug controlled by a profit-driven company with a monopoly.

When the WTO delegates met in Doha in November, they hammered out an agreement that clearly put public health interests above profit. The agreement explicitly recognized the suffering caused by AIDS, tuberculosis and malaria and it stressed that TRIPS "can and should be interpreted and implemented in a manner supportive of WTO Members' right to protect public health and, in particular, to promote access to medicines for all." The poorest countries were told they did not have to grant pharmaceutical patents until 2016. The Doha agreement also confirmed their right to manufacture or import generic versions of essential drugs, and not only during emergencies. However, the delegates could not agree about whether generic manufacturers should be able to export drugs to countries unable to make their own, since TRIPS states that compulsory licensing is intended "primarily for the supply of the domestic market." The upshot for poor countries was that their right to import cheaper drugs was effectively rendered meaningless, since other nations wouldn't be allowed to fill their orders.

The WTO members agreed to resolve the sticking point by the end of 2002. After intense negotiation they missed that deadline, but they finally reached a decision on August 30, 2003. Again, public health prevailed. The agreement allows generic manufacturers to export drugs to countries that lack the ability to produce them, provided they meet several conditions: they must openly declare these exports to the WTO, for example, and they are asked to use special packaging, coloring or shapes designed to prevent the drugs from being diverted and sold illegally in other countries. Western nations fought for even stricter controls, including limits on which diseases constituted a public health problem, but were unable to obtain them. "The final piece of the jigsaw has fallen into place," the head of the WTO boasted after the agreement, "allowing poorer countries to make full use of the flexibilities in the WTO's intellectual property rules in order to deal with the diseases that ravage their people. It proves once and for all that the organization can handle humanitarian as well as trade concerns." MSF acknowledged the progress, but remained skeptical about whether these agreements will have any teeth: "Trade rules and declarations are one thing on paper," it declared in a press release, "but they will only mean something to sick people when countries begin to put them into practice."

There were some positive signs, but just as many setbacks. In the spring of 2004, Canada became the first industrialized nation to pass a law that ostensibly allows generic manufacturers to export affordable drugs to poorer countries. The legislation was heralded as a leap forward by many observers, but not by MSF officials, who said the bill had too many limiting clauses, such as a list of eligible drugs that didn't include fixed-dose combinations for treating HIV. Meanwhile, just weeks after the August agreement, MSF accused the United States of bullying Cambodia into amending its laws to discourage the availability of generic drugs. MSF also argued that the gains made within the WTO are being undermined by regional trade deals, such as the Free Trade Areas of the Americas agreement, due to be finalized in 2005. The FTAA may force countries such as Haiti to give up their exemption from issuing patents on medicines, and it may limit compulsory licensing to national emergencies only. MSF has called the agreement "the most far-reaching and extreme attempt to weaken the Doha declaration."

MSF and its allies showed that the price of antiretrovirals could decrease by a factor of at least 30 without bankrupting pharmaceutical companies. Activists have pushed AIDS to the top of the public health agenda, and they have had the right to affordable treatment set out in international trade agreements. But with every step forward, there's always someone tugging a little harder on the leash, and doctors are still planning funerals for their patients. MSF is well aware that it can achieve only so much. "It's so much bigger than us," says Richard Bedell, "but we can't be paralyzed by the absence of a perfect solution."

8 | Best Performance in a Supporting Role

Patrick Lemieux slips off his dusty sandals, ducks his head and steps into a tiny mud-brick hut. Inside, the floor is covered with a red and blue woven carpet, and its perimeter is ringed with cushions, illuminated by the sunlight that enters through small holes in the walls. Lemieux sits down opposite two Pashtun men, one clad from turban to toe in black, the other in immaculate white. Both are elders in the community of displaced Afghans who have settled in Spin Boldak, right on the Pakistan border. A few minutes later, a man enters the hut with two steaming pots of *chai* and a plate of pink and orange sugar cubes. Lemieux turns to his translator and asks, "What gives the sugar these colors?" The Afghan nods and smiles. "Sugar!" It's clear that his English is barely a step above Lemieux's Pashto. Just then a VHF radio crackles to life and a few English words are heard over the airwaves. Lemieux takes the handset from his belt and holds it up for the elders to see. "George Bush," he says, pointing to the speaker, and they erupt in laughter.

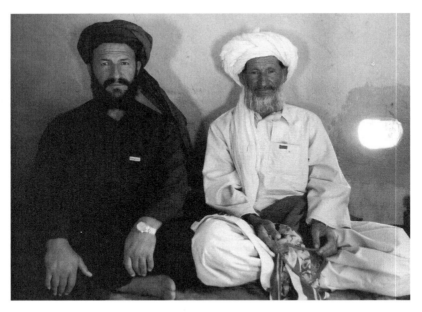

Afghan elders prepare to share chai *with MSF volunteers at a camp in Spin Boldak, on the border with Pakistan. When the organization sets up a new project, non-medical members of the team become the face of MSF in the community.*

It's a risky joke to make in Afghanistan, perhaps, but Lemieux knows what he's doing. As the acting project coordinator for MSF's team in Chaman, in southwestern Pakistan, which includes running a basic health unit at this camp for displaced people, he's doing a little public relations, trying to get the community leaders to understand the organization's role. Whether he's taking tea with elders in the camp or chatting about the Koran with Pakistani border officials, his MSF vest is often the first one the population sees. Two days later, standing in front of a whiteboard in the Chaman compound, he gives the same message to his national staff, many of whom see MSF as just another foreign organization in a region that has seen far too many of them. "We're a medical NGO working with refugees," he stresses to the locals, "not an American puppet gathering information." His concerns are not trivial – neatly painted graffiti on the outside walls of the compound attest to the anti-Western feelings in the region. Motorbikes sputter around the town flying black-and-white striped flags, the Taliban version of Jolly Rogers. For now, the team has exchanged its trademark Land Cruisers for unmarked minibuses, and there's no MSF flag over the compound, no logo on the gate.

Like Lemieux, who has a law degree and an MBA, about 40 percent of MSF's expats in the field are neither doctors nor nurses, but part of a supporting cast. Each section has a head of mission, who oversees all the projects in a given country. Project coordinators are in charge of a team's daily activities, including hiring staff and monitoring security. Financial coordinators crunch the numbers. Water and sanitation engineers sink wells and dig latrines. And logisticians do just about anything, from fixing vehicles to procuring supplies. In the jargon of aid workers, the members of this group are called PCs, fincos, watsans and logs. Then there are humanitarian affairs officers, often human rights lawyers or specialists in international relations, who advise field teams and headquarters staff about the political contexts in which they work. With all these dramatis personae sharing the stage, some in the organization feel that the balance is tipping in the wrong direction: "For me it's getting to the point where it's Doctors Without Doctors," one surgeon says wryly. Still, MSF would not be able to deliver health care without the hundreds of non-medical volunteers it sends to the field.

Chris Day started his MSF tenure as a log, despite admitting to no technical skills: "If your car breaks down, you're fucked if I'm the logistician." He's found his niche as a project coordinator, a job that requires equal amounts of administrative and diplomatic aplomb. During one mission in West Africa, he returned from a short break to find that civil war had broken out – in the team. "It was just a daily, exhausting effort to contain this conflict, and it wore me out. I remember one day being so tired that I put a CD in and lay back on the floor for a second, and when I woke up it was hours later. I just passed out because I was so tired from dealing with these people bickering, because they couldn't sit down and talk to each other. It was so petty and childish, I was so angry, and I'm still learning to deal with that kind of thing. I credit myself, to a certain extent, with being able to keep teams together. I think that's one of the skills I've developed. But you never know. The law of averages says, especially with the type of misfits that MSF attracts, in a group of ten people you're going to have one freak."

Like Lemieux, Day usually begins his missions by meeting with local bigwigs and trying to establish a rapport. "That's my job, being the face of MSF in the community, making sure everyone knows exactly what we're doing there. If the rebels and the community know me as a person, and can see tangibly what we're doing, and they like it, it increases our security." Day's mission in Ivory Coast in 2003, however, got off to a rough start. Just two days into the job, he and the head of mission were leaving an MSF hospital in the town of Man when they were caught in the middle of a gun battle. They bailed out of the car and had to hide in the grass until the ground stopped shaking. A couple of months later, Day and a colleague, Rich Zereik, paid a visit to a rebel commander named Fargass to ask about some shooting that had woken them up the night before. "Fargass was just sitting there and he said,

'Don't worry about that, it was nothing. We went to interrogate a woman, tempers rose, and people started shooting. It's no big deal. In fact, I'm disarming them this morning.' Little did we know he was disarming them *now*, right there.

"There was a curtain over the window, so we couldn't see what was going on outside, but we could hear vehicles pulling up, and I could just picture in my mind pickups full of fighters, fully armed, jumping down from the trucks. Soon there was a big, sweaty, angry mob of young men with guns outside. A lot of yelling, a lot of shoving, a lot of tempers. We were trapped in the office, and Fargass and one of his boys were walking in and out carrying hardware with them and setting it down, and slowly this mountain of guns started to appear. Rich and I are just sitting there, and Fargass is saying, 'Excuse me, I'll just be a minute.'

"The moment that terrified me was when the chief of security came in, slammed the door, and put one hand on the door and the other on his pistol. There was a moment where he collected himself – with his hand bracing the door, he looked down and took a deep breath. I thought a bunch of guys were going to just burst through the door and start shooting. And there was nowhere for us to go. Then he looked up and said, 'No, no, don't worry, we'll be with you in a minute. It's fine.' Finally, the angry crowd dispersed, and there's me and Rich still sitting there, going, 'What the fuck?' Fargass came back in, lit a cigarette, and sat down with his eyes closed. We just sat there in silence for a few minutes, and then he suddenly opened his eyes and just started talking. 'You know, I'm only twenty-seven. I've got a lot of responsibility here.' He kind of unburdened himself to us. After that, Fargass was really cool to me. It was sort of a bond – a narrow-escape-from-death bond."

Negotiating with government soldiers and rebel leaders in the field is a skill that has to be learned on the job – and relearned on every mission. "I've shaken hands with killers," says logistician Martin Girard. "It was part of my job in Colombia. We were going down the river, and we needed the permission from the paras." The paras – short for paramilitaries, and also known as the AUC – are a group of right-wing militias, financed mainly by drug money, who have been linked with some of the country's most brutal killings. "We were meeting in the office of the health secretary of the province, and this commander comes in and sits down with us. He's full of tattoos, with sixteen gold chains, and he's got death in his eyes. This guy could kill someone and go back to eating his chicken, and he wouldn't give a shit. You could see that – he had lots of marks on his gun. He'd killed lots of guys. And we had to sit down and ask this guy, politely, 'We would like to go down to this village and start a project there. Would you agree to let us take our boat down the river?' He asked if we had the green light from Carlos Castaño, the big boss of the AUC, and we said 'Yes, there's no problem.' And he said, 'If Carlos says yes, I say yes.' Top to bottom, they were very disciplined people.

"This is something that's very difficult to do with child soldiers in Sierra Leone. These kids are ten years old, drugged or drunk, trigger happy all the time. How do you control a thing like that? How do you reason with a kid like that at a checkpoint? You do it very politely. You treat him like a four-star US general. If I had a cold chain of measles vaccines worth two hundred grand in my two trucks, I had to be polite. There are moments where you really can communicate with these kids. They're very special moments, where for a few seconds they kind of go back to their childhood and forget about their guns and say, 'You're a nice guy, you treated me well.' Mind you, when you get a teenager who's been fighting for eight years in the bush, and who's really addicted to the ideology of his movement, this is trickier."

"There's an art to crossing checkpoints," agrees Peter Lorber, who did several missions as a logistician in Africa and Asia. "In Tajikistan, I was telling other expats how to approach checkpoints: take your sunglasses off, keep your hands visible. Absolutely, positively turn off every radio, hide every camera. Smile. Roll the window down halfway, but not all the way – you don't want them reaching in, but you don't want to seem like you're sealed off. If you stop, that's very scary for guys standing at a checkpoint. If you go too fast, that's also scary. It's a touchy area, so it's always good if you can get out, share some bread, give a cigarette, talk to people, let them know that you're OK. But how you approach a checkpoint in Tajikistan is different from how you approach a checkpoint in Nigeria. Every place is different, and they can't have a course on this stuff."

When agencies like MSF are given permission to work in an area, they are supposed to be able to pass through checkpoints unaccosted. But during Lorber's mission in Nigeria, soldiers often demanded money, something MSF wasn't prepared to accept. "We decided that every one of our Toyotas was going to have boxes of condoms in the glove box. So instead of giving them money at the checkpoints, we started giving out condoms, and it broke the ice. They started laughing about it: 'No, dees one too small, dees one too small!' It was consistent with MSF – we found a creative way to get around it; we didn't bribe people. That's always the best way. If you can humanize the situation, you get by."

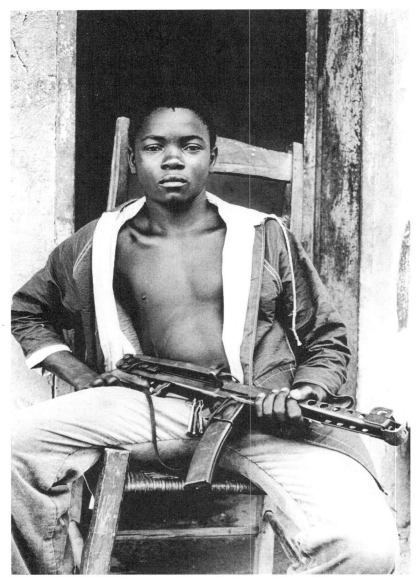

Negotiating access to patients can be difficult when checkpoints are manned by child soldiers like this one in Monrovia. Non-medical volunteers undergo a training course before their first MSF mission, but negotiation is one of the skills they have to learn on the job.

Giving out condoms is a common practice elsewhere in Africa too, one that many believe is good for both parties. But Chris Day doesn't buy that argument. "They always tried to ask us for condoms, and we just said, 'No, go to the hospital.' I refuse to give anything at checkpoints. In principle, you'd think that giving them condoms would be good, but not at checkpoints. Because we have a laissez-passer that lets us pass through checkpoints, and the minute you start giving them things it becomes a toll. When I have an emergency transfer in the car, I'm not going to stop to deal with some stoned teenager who won't let me pass until I give him a condom. I have a laissez-passer from his commander, and I will not stop just because he has a gun.

"You have to be respectful, but at the same time, you can't take shit from people. Young African men will respect that you won't take shit from them. If you're both young men, I think there's a kind of mutual understanding – you can just be young guys together and be cool with each other. Once in a while you're going to get some prick, and that's when you need to be respectful and polite. I take the piss out of them at checkpoints all the time, and they collapse in laughter, but that's only after you get to know them a bit. It's trial and error, believe me."

Peter Lorber, whose pre-MSF days were spent working as a geophysicist and a Texas fire captain, describes a logistician's role as "doing whatever needs to be done so doctors can just be doctors." Chris Day, with tongue in cheek, defines it as "dealing with an infinite series of inconsequential tasks that, at the end of the day, make you feel like you haven't accomplished anything."

During a single mission, an MSF logistician might supervise the construction of new health clinics, install radio equipment and satellite dishes, renovate the team's living quarters, find parts for a broken Land Cruiser, hire local craftsmen, book flights for expats, and find shipments of supplies that got stuck in customs. This array of responsibilities means MSF logs come from diverse backgrounds – they're mechanics, ship captains, construction workers, tree planters and tour operators. (While most other positions in MSF are filled more or less equally by both sexes, logs are overwhelmingly male.) Good logisticians know a little about a lot, and while they're not all technical wizards, they must be quick-thinking, resourceful troubleshooters, able to acclimatize swiftly in unfamiliar environments.

"You could work an entire day and not get anything done," David Croft says of his project in Kandahar. "All you do is support the medical team, or administration, or a fuse gets blown, and suddenly it's three in the afternoon and you realize you haven't even touched the long list of jobs you wanted to get done." Before Croft went to Afghanistan with MSF, he was a scuba instructor in Zanzibar, ran a safari camp in Kenya and led overland tours in Africa. "Being an overland driver teaches you to be handy – you get good at mechanics, you learn a lot about electrics, construction, fixing roads that are falling down around your vehicle. You learn about living in a closed environment with a group of strangers – and not only living with them, but also leading them, showing them a good time, dealing with their problems, making sure they're well fed when there's no food to be found, watching them have arguments and fights, and trying to maintain a positive dynamic, which can be very tricky. You cover a wide spectrum, which goes well with this job."

Despite having traveled widely, it took Croft a while to get used to Afghanistan, but he soon grew to enjoy working with his national staff. "I'd never really known an Afghan till I went there, and those guys have a fantastic sense of humor, they're constantly playing jokes on each other, so it was good fun. It is a very different culture, but you fall back on the tried and true things – just show people a lot of respect and have a sense of humor. I'm not the most culturally sensitive person, but I try to be respectful toward people, which goes a long way. It's a tough situation, because they see a lot of expats come and go, and they're always the same – they're really the glue that keeps the whole operation together. They know their jobs, and every time an expat comes along he wants to do something different. I've adapted fairly simply to them, I haven't tried to understand too much about their lives. I respect the fact that they pray five times a day, which is fine, though it tends to be when you need a car.

"It's a bit tough because you've got to know when to be firmer with them and when to just have a laugh and let things go. You don't want to cause offense, but at the same time, you're not going to let the guys take the piss out of you. There were a couple of guys who were notorious for going off and having a snooze, and I always busted them. I knew where they were snoozing, and I always had a really shitty job for them to do right after. They either took the message or they got better at hiding. Most of them were very confident, solid workers. It's just different; it's not North America or Europe. They don't put their noses to the grindstone eight hours a day. They work when there's a job to do, and when there's not, they have *chai*. And that's the way I like it."

Even if Day and Croft often felt that they hadn't accomplished much, MSF's logistics are among the best in the aid community, thanks to the organization's financial resources and three decades of experience. Nurse Leanne Olson – admittedly, she's married to a logistician – says it's one thing that sets MSF apart in the field. "When there's an emergency, MSF can be on the ground with the staff and the equipment within days. They don't have to ask for money, they don't have to piss around getting supplies and materials. They're so experienced now that they can function at a very high level, very quickly. They seem to somehow come up with who they need, what they need, when they need it. They don't always do it in the right way, they don't always do it in the most diplomatic way, but they are able to do it. In every project I've been on, if I said I need another driver, another car, another nurse, or I need to renovate this place – whatever I needed, I got. In Sierra Leone, I needed a clinic in ten days, and they built a clinic in ten days from scratch – fence, walls, buildings, wells, latrines, cleaning staff, nursing staff."

In some established projects, logisticians can find what they need locally. However, to move quickly in an emergency, MSF uses prepacked medical kits that can be quickly shipped from warehouses to anywhere in the world within about 48 hours. Two of MSF's logistical centers – one near Bordeaux, the other in northern Belgium – also supply these kits to other aid agencies. Although every crisis is unique, natural disasters and disease outbreaks have many predictable elements. Responding to an earthquake, for example, a team may order several disaster kits, each of which contains medical supplies

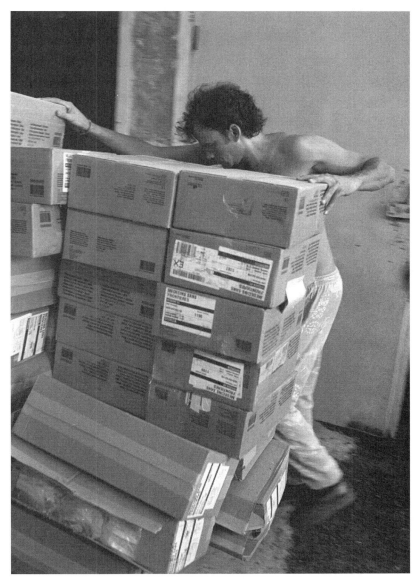

An MSF team unloads 20 tons of supplies that will go to support a mission in Georgia, in the North Caucasus. The logisticians who arrange shipments like this toil outside the media spotlight, but their work is a crucial part of any medical project.

to treat a thousand slightly wounded people in a health clinic with no doctor. If there is a cholera outbreak in a refugee camp, cholera kit 001 contains everything you need to treat 625 patients: oral rehydration salts, IV infusions, disinfectant, water chlorination supplies, even the pens, pencils and stationery. To make it easier to arrange air transport, the catalog lists the volume and weight of the kits – a disaster kit weighs 600 pounds, a cholera kit more than 13,000 – and lists any drugs that need to be kept cool or require special handling. In addition to these medical toolboxes, there are prepacked communications kits (radios and handsets, for example), water and sanitation kits and catalogs full of individual supplies, from inkjet printers to latrine squat plates.

But even the most well-provisioned logistician can't anticipate every problem, as Lorber found when he set up a refrigeration system in a hospital in the former Soviet republic of Azerbaijan. MSF was running a drug distribution program in the area, and Lorber needed to establish a cold chain, making sure vaccines were kept at the right temperature as they were transported. "You do the best you can building the refrigerators and the freezers – some things need deep freeze, some things need refrigeration – and I went through battle after battle. I got a dedicated electric line from the military to this clinic where we were going to start the immunization, because the local electricity was working only an hour or two a day. Even then, it could be anywhere from eighty to three hundred volts on a different day, and I couldn't put in good enough stabilizers to prevent the fridges from getting fried. So I bought a case of champagne for the military commander, I got a dedicated electric line to my cold storage, put in all the refrigerators and put in these devices that electronically record temperature history. I was satisfied, and we got the vaccines in. The next day I went back to check on it, and the vaccines were in a pile on the floor, and inside the fridge were bottles of vodka, Fanta orange soda and a sheep's head that belonged to the director of the hospital. The vaccines were already spoiled. What do you do? Sometimes you yell, sometimes you laugh."

MSFers who handle the money – and in some projects, this can be considerable sums of cash – also have to understand and navigate the local economy. "Corruption is not just an evil little footnote," says Lorber. "In lots of places in the world, corruption *is* the economy. So you're really not doing yourself any favors if you jump into a place and you've got a self-righteous attitude." He admits to using some creative negotiating to get medical cargo through customs urgently, although that technique backfired on him in Uganda. "I was trying to clear some IV fluids and the customs office at Entebbe was about to close for three days. There was a seething mass of people trying to get in, and I was fighting to get to the front. I finally got up to this customs official and offered him some money, and he was so profoundly offended. He stood up, he started yelling at me: What did I think he was? Imagine you're doing your job the best you can in a place that's struggling and a bit broken down, and somebody insults your principles by offering you money."

In many developing countries, aid organizations are major employers of local people, and they bring a great deal of money into the economy. Nabil al-Tikriti, who has worked as an MSF administrator in five countries, admits to wondering whether that money sometimes greases the wrong hands, perhaps even perpetuating the corruption. During his first MSF project in Kismayu, Somalia, in 1993, his job included paying about 120 local employees. He would give a bundle of Somali cash to an assistant, who would dole it out to the staff – the currency was so devalued that each person received a sack of bills. Then one man, who had a connection to one of the local warlords, would take a cut from all the others. "It was a rudimentary taxation system – he would hit them up for one wad of cash out of their twenty. What he did with it we were not allowed to find out. I was burning through something like forty thousand dollars a month in cash, and that was all going straight into that economy. Now forty thousand isn't a grand amount, really, but there was so little happening in Kismayu that we really wondered what our effect on the war economy was. We had the most valuable items around, and we did get ripped off a couple of times. The economy had so little going on that we were kind of the only game in town. I have to admit, at the time I didn't think much of it, because it was something that the entire staff expected. Nobody complained about it."

If there are any unsung heroes in MSF, they must surely be the water, sanitation and hygiene specialists. While the media spotlight shines on doctors and nurses, there are no admiring throngs around the pumps and wells, no TV closeups of sharps-disposal containers, and no one strewing rose petals in the path of the trucks that empty latrines. Yet in areas where diarrheal diseases are a leading cause of death, or where mosquito-borne malaria is rampant, watsans can be the bringers of life.

MSF water and sanitation projects are usually emergency relief efforts, such as treating an epidemic among refugees, or part of a larger program, such as building a new health center. Watsans make sure that the clinics and hospitals they support have an adequate water supply, that waste is disposed of safely, and that proper infection controls are in place. They design isolation wards, ensuring they're properly ventilated, and check that people can move through with minimal risk. Their work may also have an epidemiological component, as they track the origin of a cholera outbreak or the breeding patterns of mosquitoes. "Some organizations do water for water's sake," says Liz Walker, a watsan adviser with the Belgian section, "because as well as health benefits, there are also socioeconomic benefits. But MSF is really looking to target specific diseases, or certain problems based on data we've collected from our medical programs."

Walker was educated as a civil engineer in England, where she spent several years in industry, but a volunteer stint in Tanzania made it clear that her UK training was "next to useless" in Africa. She returned home to get a master's degree, specializing in water technologies in developing countries. A year after graduation, she found herself in rural Tibet, where scores of small villages were plagued with diarrhea, scabies and eye infections. "The villages were generally on the valley floor, and they would usually fetch their water from way up in the hills, but more and more people were drinking water from the irrigation channels, which, of course, are highly polluted."

MSF set about to catch the clean water from springs up in the hills and pipe it down to reservoirs in the villages. Walker's team would begin by locating the eye of the spring – the place where it emerges from the ground – because, once it reaches the surface, it's no longer pristine. "What you want to do is narrow it down to a small point, so you can capture it and protect it from contamination. In rock, you'll usually see it come out of the ground only in one place, whereas in mixed ground you have to dig down to rock. You might see it come up in four or five places, and you have to chase the water down six or eight meters. You can cut half the hillside away." Once the source was located, the crew would roll several miles of polyethylene pipe into the yard-deep trenches the villagers had dug. These pipes led to a reservoir in the village, which in turn fed several taps from which the villagers filled their containers. During the icy Tibetan winter, the water between the springs and the reservoirs did not freeze because the pipes were buried deeply enough. "But between the reservoir and the taps, and where the taps are coming up to the surface, it would indeed freeze, so in the winter they would make one guy responsible for draining that system every night and refilling it every morning. Usually the guy would forget once, but after that the village would make sure he never forgot again."

Walker later coordinated a similar project in Rwanda, bringing water from springs into the MSF health center, with taps installed at intervals along the way for the community. "You can't supply just the hospital, or the population will come along and dig up your pipe." When she worked in Sudan, MSF flew around with 5 tons of drilling equipment and sunk boreholes every hundred yards to bring groundwater to the people. In these cases, the water is pure when it arrives at the taps or the hand pumps, but it can still get contaminated when it's carried in an unwashed bucket or a filthy jerry can, so watsans treat it with a residual chlorine that continues to act even after the water is removed from the source. In areas where people are drinking from rivers and streams, in some cases even swamps, it's more complicated. Most rivers in Africa are turbid – clouded with sediment – and chlorination isn't enough. To clarify the water, technicians use a method called coagulation and flocculation, in which a chemical such as aluminum sulfate causes the particles to coalesce and sink to the bottom. Then the clear water is taken off the top and treated with chlorine. "That is something we would do in an emergency," Walker explains, "and MSF would provide all the chemicals. But in community projects you try to find water that is pure at source, because chemical treatment is not something the community can continue with."

In 2000, after an explosion of malaria in the Great Lakes region of Africa, Walker helped launch an entirely different type of watsan project, one that had nothing to do with drinking water. MSF targeted a number of villages in Burundi with a high elevation, close to the upper limit of where *Anopheles* mosquitoes can live. When local farmers began to grow new crops there, including rice, the number of malaria cases rose dramatically. "Paddy fields provide a fantastic breeding ground for mosquitoes. So in the highlands of Burundi and elsewhere – Kenya, Rwanda, Uganda – you've got these high-level plateaus where the mosquitoes have managed to get a foothold at a higher elevation than they were used to." Those mosquitoes brought malaria into an area where it had been uncommon, and even adults began dying because they had little or no immunity. Walker helped launch a "vector control" program that treated the houses adjacent to the breeding sites with residual insecticide. "The hope is that this will act as a barrier to the houses above. Mosquitoes don't fly that far, and those that do would be killed en route. We tackled thirteen thousand households, which is only about ten percent, but we hope it will have a much larger impact in the province – by providing this barrier, you're protecting everyone else."

As in purely medical projects, the challenges in watsan

activities are not just technical but cultural. Diseases don't disappear as soon as clean water comes out of the taps, so teams include a hygiene promoter, often an expat, who looks at people's practices and attitudes and identifies the biggest risk factors. Do people wash their hands after going to the latrine? Are they using dirty water containers? Are they bathing children properly? MSF usually targets certain groups – say, mothers or children – and, depending on literacy levels and the media available, staff members speak on the radio, hand out leaflets or create a series of drawings that model good habits. "We're often working with schools," Walker says. "In the Rwanda project, the kids were asked to make up a drama about hygiene. The best classes from each school competed against each other, and we found that to be very effective. Nearly everybody we questioned had heard about this competition or gone to see it. Sometimes we have drama groups going around with specific messages, or we have songs or quizzes. We have a hygiene snakes and ladders game – if they answer the questions right, they shoot up the ladder, and if they answer wrong, they shoot down the snake."

Sometimes the political context is a factor, too. Tibetans have lived for decades under a Communist system in which the state owns, and ostensibly maintains, all the infrastructure. As a result, Walker says, villagers are sometimes reluctant to take personal responsibility for looking after their new water system. (In the larger picture, MSF withdrew from Tibet altogether in 2003 because it was unable to work within the Chinese public health system.) "On the other hand, when you try to mobilize people to do community work, the response is astounding. Hundreds of people would turn up to dig trenches – they'd just say, 'OK, where do you want them?' and off they go. Some of these systems were several kilometers long, and everyone would go out and dig a few meters. They wouldn't even think to say, 'How about a salary?'"

Walker was also surprised to find that the villagers and MSF weren't necessarily piping in water for the same reasons. "For us, it's health we're pushing, and we're doing education at the same time: 'Drink safe water, wash your hands,' etcetera. But Tibetans have a thousand and one reasons they wanted fresh water, and health may well not be on their list. When we finished a project, we'd have an inauguration, a big ceremony, and the people would invariably come and ply me with beer for hours and hours, and thank me, and that's when we heard what they got out of it. The women had been going three or five kilometers into the hills to carry this water, so for them it was about saving time and effort. Then there was a group of teenaged lads who came to express their thanks with much nudge-nudge, wink-wink, and shuffling of feet. Their perception of the benefit was that all the women in the valley now wanted to live in their village, so their wedding prospects had just multiplied tenfold."

A water engineer might call that a trickle-down effect.

9 | New Fridge Syndrome

Kenny Gluck knew something was up when he saw a car slide out from the roadside to block the convoy he was traveling in. "We had left the hospital in four vehicles, and we hadn't even gotten out of the town yet when two cars cut us off – one in the front, one in the back – and a bunch of people in masks and carrying Kalashnikovs got out." The men opened fire, but no one was hit – their goal wasn't to kill but to scare. "And they succeeded," Gluck says dryly. "They pulled me out of our car and pushed me into theirs. They whacked me over the head with a rifle butt and then put a coat over my head so I couldn't see."

It was January 9, 2001, and Gluck, 38 at the time, was MSF-Holland's head of mission for the North Caucasus, which includes war-torn Chechnya. On the day he was abducted, Gluck was leaving the town of Stariye Atagi, about 12 miles from the Chechen capital of Grozny. It's an area he knows well, having worked in Chechnya from 1994 to 1996 with another NGO, and since early 2000 with MSF. He's

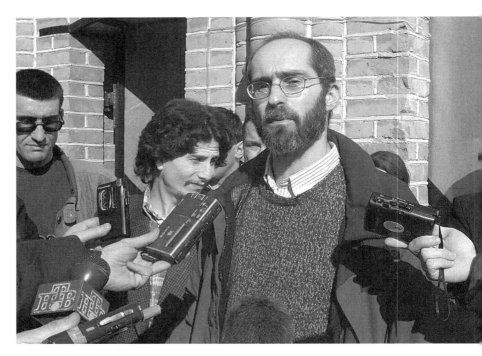

Kenny Gluck speaks to the media three days after he was freed by his captors in Chechnya. As head of mission for the Dutch section, Gluck was abducted in January 2001 and held for almost a month. No ransom was demanded, and the identity of the kidnappers is still unknown.

fluent in Russian, too, though it didn't help him that day in the kidnappers' car. "They didn't say anything except, 'Shut up and keep your head down.' We drove for about an hour, switched cars, then they put me in a house where we waited for a while." Gluck was moved three times that first night, before being forced into the root cellar of another house. The floorboards were just a few feet above him, making it difficult to sit up. Onions, cabbages and carrots lay on the rocky dirt floor, along with a mattress that would be Gluck's bed for the next nine nights.

Kidnapping is something of a national pastime in Chechnya, and expats are not exempt from the violence. In 1995, veteran aid worker Fred Cuny visited Chechnya on behalf of billionaire philanthropist George Soros, only to disappear in April. It's assumed he was murdered, along with three colleagues, though their bodies have never been found. The following year, six Red Cross workers – four Europeans, a Canadian and a New Zealander – were sleeping in their hospital compound, not far from where Gluck was abducted, when they were executed by masked men carrying guns fitted with silencers. Then Camilla Carr and Jon James, British psychologists working with a small Quaker NGO, were abducted in July 1997 and held for 14 months. By the time Carr and James were released, MSF had pulled out of Chechnya because of the insecurity, but by February 2000 they were back. And so were the kidnappings – that August three more Red Cross workers were abducted, though they were released after a week. In all, at least 50 humanitarian aid workers have been kidnapped in the North Caucasus since 1996.

Finding those responsible for these attacks is extremely difficult. To begin with, the abductors do not usually make ransom demands; often there is no negotiation at all. The region's power politics are complex – Gluck estimates there are 50 or 60 active military groups, and their alliances are rarely clear. So, when he was dragged from the car and MSF received no communication from his attackers, the trail quickly turned cold. The organization immediately suspended all its activities in the area and called on the Russian authorities to investigate, but even Gluck himself didn't know why he was being held. "They talked to me quite a bit, but I didn't feel that the people talking to me were the decision makers; they were just guards. They said they were hoping to trade me for captured people, but I don't know if that was true. They were Chechens, I could tell that, but I didn't know whether they were fighting on the Russian side or the anti-Russian side. I didn't get to those questions."

Gluck's case is proof that the best type of security is being known in the community. "All the Chechen doctors there knew me, and I had a lot of friends in this area, and they were getting in touch with everybody – Russian groups, criminal groups, pro-Chechen groups – saying this was unacceptable. People who deal in these activities get wounded a lot, so the Chechen surgeons had operated on a lot of people, and they just went to all their contacts and started pushing for my release. To each of the groups they thought could be involved they would say, 'Look, your mother or your cousin was treated in an MSF-built surgical facility, with MSF drugs that Kenny himself brought in here. How can you do this? You have to take responsibility for getting him out.' Partly they were saying unethical things, like, 'We're going to stop treating your people if this keeps going on.'

"My conditions improved dramatically after that first nine or ten days, and I'm pretty sure that around this time some of these doctors got lucky and talked to the right group. Someone was getting through to the kidnappers and saying, 'Treat him nicely.' After that, I was moved to a room that was about two meters by a meter and a half. They surprised me – they came and asked what kind of food I wanted, what I needed. I didn't ask for any change in the food – I thought it was fine before. They were just giving me normal Chechen village food, nothing surprising, and more than enough of it. What I said was, I need news, things to read, and they gave me that."

A few days after he was moved from the cellar, Gluck's captors assured him he had nothing to fear. "According to them it was settled, and it was just a matter of working out how I would be released. I was talking with them a lot about how to do it, and in the end they did exactly as I requested." He suggested that the kidnappers drop him off at the home of a Chechen surgeon who was a personal friend of his as well as being known among both the separatist and the pro-Russian groups. But the days dragged on and he began to wonder if it was false hope. "Things happened that were terrifying – there were moments when I thought they were taking me outside to shoot me. There were times when the house shook so hard from the shelling that plaster was falling off the walls."

Finally, on the night of February 4, Gluck was told he was going to be freed. They put a mask over his head and bundled him out of the house and into a car. "In the car they were very apologetic. These were different people – by their voices, I could tell these were older people, clearly with more authority. They were apologizing to MSF, saying, 'This group didn't know who you were, we're very sorry, we're going to punish them,' all of that. While I was blindfolded, they gave me back my passport. I had passes from the Russian military to travel in Chechnya, and they gave me those back, as well as my MSF ID card. I'd had seven hundred dollars in cash in my pocket, because we needed to make some advances on construction material, and they gave me that, which surprised me a lot. I'd had a very cheap watch which I always carried – you know, seven dollars on Canal Street in New York – and they said, 'We're really sorry, we can't find your watch.' I was like, 'I'll live.'"

Around midnight, the mystery voices stopped the car and pushed Gluck out. He asked whether he could remove the blindfold, but they refused, telling him simply to walk away from the car. Then they drove off. "I heard someone yelling at me in Chechen, so I said, 'I don't speak Chechen, speak to me in Russian.' And he said in a very crude way, 'Who the hell are you?' I lifted off the mask and I realized it was the Chechen surgeon." Gluck's liberators had driven him right into the doctor's compound. "He yelled at his wife, 'Get up! We have a guest. Put food on the table.'"

Immediately, the Russian secret service, the FSB, took credit for securing Gluck's release, but it soon became clear that claim was nonsense. The Russian authorities had been as ineffective as they usually are when aid workers are abducted. MSF says it doesn't know exactly who was responsible for the kidnapping or the release, but before Gluck was pushed from the car, the liberators placed a letter in his hand. It was an apology from Shamil Basayev, the one-legged Chechen commander who, in 2002, would claim responsibility for the hostage-taking at a Moscow theater that ended in the death of some 170 people. But Basayev did not say that his people were responsible for the abduction – only that he had used his authority to secure Gluck's release. "He said it wasn't one of his groups, otherwise it wouldn't have happened, and that, because we were providing medical care in this area, he had ordered that nobody touch us, and that we were not seen as anti-Chechen. Is that a statement of responsibility or not? It's kind of vague. And I can't go back and ask them because I never saw them. All I know is the voices."

If there's one thing that annoys MSFers more than being asked why they do humanitarian aid work, it's being asked whether they're afraid of getting killed. Many downplay the risks, arguing that traffic accidents or avoidable acts of stupidity kill more aid workers than landmines or gun-toting rebels. "I'm more worried when I drive through the south side of Chicago than any other place I've been on earth," says surgeon Bruce Frank. "People get really paranoid about the safety thing. They have wild imaginations about going to different countries and how dangerous it is, when in fact there's no real palpable danger." That's not quite true, of course, but MSFers agree that the work always seems less dangerous when they're actually there doing it. Curfews and guidelines give them a sense of security, false or otherwise. Sometimes there's so much to do in a health clinic or a feeding center that there's no time to worry about rumors that the rebels are in town. Experienced volunteers get a feel for the situation in their area, and violence even a few miles away doesn't feel threatening. Meanwhile, friends and family back home often paint entire countries – or in the case of Africa, an entire continent – with the same blood-stained brush. Are you sure you want to be in Kinshasa, they ask, when there's violence in Bunia? It's like worrying about walking the streets of Tulsa because Detroit has a high murder rate.

The perception of the danger is also amplified because people are sympathetic to aid workers, just as they are to police officers and firefighters. Because these professions involve personal risk in the service of others, deaths and injuries among their members make headlines more often than those of loggers, fishermen or miners, all of whom do more dangerous work. Just what is the risk of an aid worker being killed on the job? It's impossible to know for sure because there are no comprehensive statistics. While the UN and the Red Cross keep records of casualties among their staff, many other agencies, including MSF, do not – or at least they do not make them public. Some researchers have tried to analyze the available information, however. One study, published in the *British Medical Journal* in 2000, examined 375 deaths of humanitarian aid workers, both nationals and expats, between 1985 and 1998. It found that 68 percent were the result of intentional violence, such as being shot, bombed or setting off a mine; only 17 percent were motor vehicle accidents; and the average age of expats killed was 40 years – hardly greenhorns making careless mistakes. While this study confirmed that the number of deaths is rising – a commonly held belief in the aid community – it points out that the number of humanitarian aid workers in the field is also increasing, so there's no way of knowing whether the work has become statistically riskier. A more recent survey, by Dennis King of the US government's Humanitarian Information Unit, looked at reported deaths of aid workers between 1997 and 2001. He also found that violence was the leading cause – almost half the non-accidental deaths came during ambushes on vehicles by bandits or rebels.

Aid workers are also at risk for malaria, typhoid, even HIV. But these illnesses, along with landmines, plane crashes and stray bullets, are occupational hazards that MSF volunteers are prepared to confront. (In case they're blissfully unaware of the risks, they're asked to sign a daunting waiver before leaving on mission.) What they're far less willing to accept is the trend to target aid workers specifically, singling them out for abduction or even execution. Isolated incidents of this type have occurred for decades, but in recent years they've become much more common, particularly in Iraq, Afghanistan and the North

Caucasus, though in each of these regions the dynamics are different. In Iraq, where both the UN and the Red Cross offices were targeted by suicide bombers in 2003, many in the aid community believe that agencies – even the rigorously neutral Red Cross – are being targeted because they're seen as tools of the occupying coalition army. And they believe this image is the result of a deliberate strategy by the US and British governments. When Colin Powell talks about NGOs being "such an important part of our combat team," and Tony Blair says that "this war has three dimensions: the military, the political and the humanitarian one," they reinforce the idea that aid organizations are their partners rather than independent actors. In Afghanistan, the attacks – including the one that killed five MSFers in June 2004 – are usually carried out by remnants of the ousted Taliban regime who hope to scare international agencies out of the country for good. And they've had some success – many organizations have scaled back their activities. The Taliban initially won support by exploiting Afghans' fears and insecurities in the 1990s, and their only chance of returning to power depends on whether they can destabilize the country and its transitional government – something that's much easier to do without pesky aid agencies around to deliver health care and normalize people's lives. By December 2003, attacks on aid workers were averaging one a day.

"The United States has had military people on the ground who dress in T-shirts and drive around in white Land Cruisers," says Kenny Gluck. "What are they trying to do? It seems to us that they're trying to imitate aid workers, and that deliberately tries to make Afghans think [aid workers] might be soldiers. It's muddying the waters in which we have to work. The Americans want us to be their allies, and we don't want to be, because that's the death of humanitarianism if we become the allies of the American military. They want the Islamic militants to demonize us, to see us as enemies, and we have to develop the capacity to go to whoever does these attacks in Afghanistan, whether its ex-Taliban or whatever, and say 'We're not allies of the Americans. We're not even trying to rebuild this country. We're just trying to keep people alive and alleviate suffering while you and the Americans sort this out. At a fundamental level, we don't care whether bin Laden or George Bush is in charge here. It's none of our business.' And this is what other NGOs and the UN find difficult about us. A lot of other NGOs talk about the need for reconstruction – well, I don't want to be engaged in reconstruction, because I don't want Mr. Taliban to think I'm trying to rebuild his country as part of the US strategy. I want to be able to go to him honestly and say, 'All we're trying to do is keep people alive, to provide medical care for people who are wounded or sick. We're not trying to build your country at all, that's not our job.'"

In the North Caucasus, the Russian government has been accused of undermining humanitarian aid as well, but for different reasons. Chechen separatists and Russian forces have been clashing on and off since 1994, and the army has killed tens of thousands of civilians in its attempts to regain control over the region. Vladimir Putin's government is not anxious to have these events witnessed by the prying eyes of international organizations. "By working in Chechnya, we are pouring salt onto Russia's most painful wound," says MSF-Switzerland's head of mission in Russia. The government has a vested interest in seeing that insecurity keeps NGOs out, and kidnappings and murders of aid workers are effective ways to do that. There's no proof that Russian authorities have ever ordered or carried out any of these attacks themselves, although some in MSF quietly suggest that's a possibility. Whatever the case, the Russians have certainly exploited the incidents, repeatedly citing them as proof that the region is too dangerous to work in. "The Russians have created the insecurity," Gluck says. "Before I was kidnapped, a Russian general went on TV and called MSF 'spies and enemies of Russia.' Very helpful. They deliberately undermine our security by actions like that, and by not respecting independent humanitarian action. They've never come to us with any evidence, or even suggestions, that it's true. They just throw it out in the press, so we see it as a strategy to delegitimize us in the eyes of the armed factions. We think they've put us in danger."

Despite that danger, MSF continued to work in the North Caucasus after Gluck's release, and on August 12, 2002, the organization was targeted again. Arjan Erkel, a Dutch national working as the head of mission for the Swiss section, was abducted in Makhachkala, capital of the Russian republic of Dagestan, which shares a border with Chechnya. No group came forth to take responsibility. Six months after the kidnapping, with no word on whether Erkel was even alive, his young sister Rosalie made a poignant video appeal on the Web for people to sign a petition calling for the Russian authorities to step up their perfunctory investigation; the petition eventually received hundreds of thousands of signatures.

The case was immediately suspicious, leading MSF to question whether it was more than simply the work of criminals. Two members of the Russian FSB witnessed the abduction but did not intervene. The abductors must also have passed through several checkpoints to take Erkel out of Makhachkala, and they seem to have done so without difficulty. As for why the secret

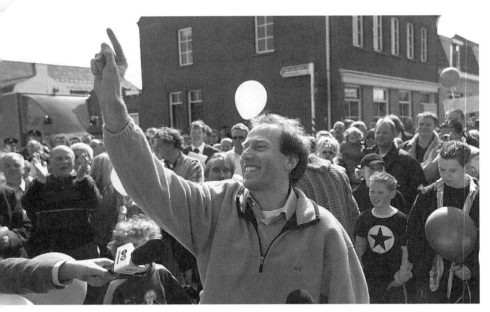

Arjan Erkel waves to supporters after arriving home in Westdorpe, the Netherlands. Erkel was kidnapped while working with MSF's Swiss section in Dagestan, near war-torn Chechnya. After 607 days in captivity, during which he lost 40 pounds, he was finally released on April 11, 2004.

service was keeping a humanitarian worker under surveillance in the first place, the Dutch newspaper NRC *Handelsblad* reported: "The FSB of Dagestan took an interest in Erkel after he treated two American military observers to a dinner earlier that week."

On several occasions, MSF received photos and videotapes via Russian authorities, proving that Erkel was still alive and that investigators were in contact with his abductors, but no progress was made. In February 2003, more than 50 calls were billed to Erkel's mobile telephone. MSF gave these numbers to Russian authorities so they could track them but were told that "no information was obtained that would be of operational interest." Justifiably frustrated, MSF in July enlisted the help of the Veterans of Foreign Intelligence, a group of ex-KGB agents that had been recommended by a friend of the Erkel family. The veterans clearly had the ear of the abductors, and by December the group announced that they had agreed on a date and terms for Erkel's release. "Then they suddenly announced that it was not possible anymore," Jean-Hervé Bradol of MSF-France later told the Paris newspaper *Le Monde*. "We then broke off negotiations with them."

For the duration of the kidnapping, MSF criticized not only the Russian and Dagestani authorities for failing to resolve the case, but also the Dutch government for its failure to protect one of its citizens. But not wanting to jeopardize the negotiations, MSF kept its frustration out of the press. Then on March 9, 2004 – Erkel's 34th birthday – MSF received news that he was suffering from a lung infection and that his abductors were threatening to execute him. The organization finally set diplomacy aside: "We are not facing an isolated group of kidnappers hiding in the forest," Bradol told *Le Monde*. "We affirm that local and federal members of the Russian administration are involved in the negotiations and are taking advantage of it."

A month later, in the wee hours of Sunday, April 11, the veterans' organization called to say that Erkel was free and waiting to be picked up in Dagestan. MSF immediately dispatched a team to meet him, and later that day Erkel stepped out of a car in Moscow to speak to reporters. He now sported a beard and was 40 pounds lighter, but appeared in good health. "I want to thank the Lord that on this day, Easter day, he brought me back to life again. I feel fantastic. If I was in Rotterdam right now, I would kiss the floor." He hugged the leader of the veterans' group and thanked him for his help in securing the release. Meanwhile, Russian state television completely ignored the news.

How exactly the Veterans of Foreign Intelligence managed to free Erkel, even after it supposedly had stopped working for MSF, still isn't clear. Not surprisingly, no one wanted to discuss whether there was a ransom, for fear of putting other aid workers in danger. But on May 29, 2004, *Le Monde* broke the story that the Netherlands foreign affairs ministry, in a deal apparently brokered by the Kremlin, paid a million euros for Erkel's freedom. The Dutch then demanded that MSF reimburse the money, which it described as an "advance." According to the Paris newspaper, officials at MSF perceived the demand as blackmail: pay up, quickly and quietly, or we'll stop funding you. (The Dutch government, no doubt still stinging from MSF's criticism of its inaction, has been a major donor to MSF-Holland.)

For its part, MSF claims that the Dutch negotiators called "at the last minute" to say an arrangement was in the offing, but the group insists it never agreed to a loan. "They said, 'Look, there's an action going ahead, do you agree to green-light it? It's going to cost this amount of money,'" said Rowan Gillies, MSF's international president, after the story made worldwide news in June. "We said, 'We can't give you any sort of OK for the money, but certainly go ahead. We want to get him out.'" By July, however, with the dispute still unsettled, the Dutch government took the radical step of suing the Swiss section of MSF, Erkel's employer at the time of the kidnapping; the case opened on April 21, 2005, in Geneva and dragged on into the fall without resolution. Meanwhile, Erkel's kidnappers remain at large.

The whole episode was an enormous disappointment for MSF, since it makes resuming work in the region all the more dangerous. "Something like this traumatizes the whole organization," Kenny Gluck said while Erkel was still in captivity. "It forces you to question whether we should be there. Certainly a lot of people, following my kidnapping, said MSF has to leave the area. But it just feels too rotten to walk away."

Most MSF volunteers are never abducted or physically assaulted, but they all know someone who has been. Many have their own stories about close calls, moments when they thought their number was up. They may have witnessed atrocities, or at least their aftermath, and all have seen tremendous suffering from disease, famine and war. Here, too, they have a tendency to play down the psychological stress of the job, for a number of reasons. To begin with, it becomes normal very quickly. First-time volunteers often say they were amazed how quickly they became accustomed to hearing gunfire and shelling. The fear kept them awake at first, then the noise became simply an annoyance, and finally it didn't faze them at all. MSFers also tend to resent the image people have of them working in blood up to their ankles, with bullets whizzing past their heads. Certainly that's not the whole story – for many, it's not even part of the picture. No doubt there's some denial, an unwillingness to acknowledge that they're not always in control, because people can't work in an environment where they constantly feel vulnerable. But this work can take an emotional toll, even on those who thrive on the high stress and danger of insecure areas.

The aid community is not the military, and there's usually no stigma attached to people who can't take the heat – at least not any more. "Ten years ago," says Lloyd Cederstrand, "MSF had a reputation of being, I don't want to say a cowboy agency, but one with stories of surgeons going illegally to Afghanistan during the Soviet occupation, with donkeys, taking three days to get in, and doing surgery in a cave and being out of contact – they didn't have satellite phones in those days. So you almost had to be the type of person who was going to say, 'I'm going to put myself way out there, and I could be there for months.' There was a bit of that mentality. You just came back and it was, 'I've been through this, but I'm OK.' Now it's a very different climate." Cederstrand was a member of MSF-Holland's emergency team, which does short-term missions during acute crises in highly dangerous areas, such as in Liberia in the summer of 2003. Shortly after he arrived there, he saw a young boy get shot through the jaw less than a hundred feet from him, and a stray bullet struck a tree not 10 feet away. Later in the mission, a boy soldier strafed the ground in front of the MSF car. In a previous project in Somalia, Cederstrand worked with a midwife who had a soldier put a pistol to her head and pull the trigger. The gun didn't go off – only the soldier knows whether it misfired or the chamber was empty – but that was the end of the midwife's mission. MSF-Holland's psychosocial team of professional counselors, on call for just such events, immediately flew out to meet with her, and she was eventually evacuated to Amsterdam, where the organization makes longer-term counseling available.

Techniques for coping with stress are covered in the prep course taken by first-time volunteers, and senior field staff get further training in stress management, including recognizing the signs in others. In addition to teams of professionals that respond to serious incidents in the field, some sections also have less formal "peer support networks" made up of experienced volunteers who are matched with first-timers. They'll talk on the phone before the mission and again afterward, as often as needed. When volunteers have a difficult mission, they soon recognize that even the most supportive friend or family member can never really understand what they're going through, and they need to speak to someone with first-hand field experience. The model isn't perfect – "I didn't want to just talk on the phone with a stranger a couple hundred miles away," says one logistician – but it's an attempt to deal with an issue that has, until recently, been mostly ignored.

Leanne Olson, who is part of a peer support network, recognizes that there is still some reluctance on the part of volunteers to acknowledge that the stress may be getting to them. Even if they've never experienced a traumatic incident, the cumulative effect of months and years of aid work erodes people gradually. "I still think we have this macho atmosphere – we're invincible, we're heroic, we're aid workers, we can go anywhere and do anything. Because so many strong personalities end up working for MSF – it's a risky job and people don't do it if they don't like high-risk things – I think they assume that because you're pretty tough, pretty strong, you can sort yourself out. 'You know your own limits, so just don't go there.' But you don't always know your own limits, and you don't always know you've gone over them. You don't always notice that you haven't slept well in two weeks, or you've lost fifteen kilos, or you've gone from drinking a beer at dinner to drinking two, and then a whisky after that."

Drinking, and less often drugs, are ways that some MSFers deal with anxiety or boredom in the field. One project coordinator recalls how it snuck up on him during a difficult mission in West Africa. "We weren't getting hammered every night and waking up hung over every morning, but we were drinking just a little more than we should have been. Just enough to go to bed buzzed. There was nothing else to do. Then days become weeks, weeks become months. I raised the issue with my head of mission; I said, 'Look, you need to talk to people about the drinking. And I'm not excluded from this. I'm just as guilty as everyone else, and in fact, I think I'm the ringleader. But we need to think of substitutes for beer in the fridge.'"

Despite the efforts to help volunteers readjust to life at home, some feel that MSF has a tendency to fill its vacancies without enough thought to whether people are ready for another mission. Olson recalls rereading her journals one day and being surprised how many positive experiences she had written about, because only the negative ones were top of mind. "You need time to reflect on what was good, as well as what was bad. Because if you don't get rid of the bad before you go on your next mission, you take it all with you. I think a lot of people go on their next mission too quickly, without having had a chance to decompress at home. They're home for two weeks, then they're off on another mission. No, take a month, take six weeks, take the summer. Take some time to reconnect with your family and friends, get your energy back. There's always this shortage of people, and they're always saying, 'Are you ready to go yet?' and it's hard to say no. And the more experienced you are, the more they push you."

An experienced nonmedical volunteer is even more blunt. "That's where MSF is really terrible – it doesn't seem to care about the people that work for it. That's my main criticism of the organization. They could give a shit about me, man – they squeeze me like a lemon, throw me over their shoulder and then come begging for me to work when they need somebody. They don't actually try and work on people, and try to develop them. Maybe a bit, but it all depends on the crony networks you cultivate while you're in the office." Several volunteers complain that high turnover in the operational sections means they are often briefed before their departure by a person who is no longer there at the end of the mission. They come back bursting with things to say, whether about the project or about their own experiences, and feel they're met with indifference by the organization that sent them there.

Of course, the people who continue to go on mission year after year don't do it because they're being shoved onto planes by MSF headquarters. The decision is their own, but at some point it may be more about inertia, about escaping the alternatives, than about actively choosing the lifestyle. "I was joking with someone from MSF-France the other day," says a humanitarian affairs officer. "She was about forty, and she said, 'You know, I've been doing this for twelve years.' And I was telling her that I think when you pass a certain age, you're just bound to MSF. There are people who have certain ambitions, they say, 'I'm thirty-four, I want to have a kid, I want to live in a certain place, I want a better salary.' But then it's 'I don't really need a kid, I don't really need a house,' and then they're thirty-eight, thirty-nine, and then it's MSF for the rest of their life."

"You do see people who stay too long," Cederstrand agrees. "They think, 'I'm past that point, I can't settle down now, I can't have children, so I'll just keep doing this.' And you can see people are burned out, tired, who should not necessarily stop doing the work, but should stop doing it in the field. Some people realize it too late. People have mental breakdowns, and agencies don't like to talk about it. They don't like to recognize that they have people who can crash. I've seen it myself in the field, I've seen colleagues who have crashed, and it's a long recovery, because then they're forced to be back in their home society."

One might think that home, around people you care about, is exactly where you would want to recover from field-induced stress. On the contrary, most volunteers say it's much easier to leave for a mission than it is to come home. "MSF does a good job of preparing people to go somewhere," says Peter Lorber, "and you do yourself, automatically. You think, OK, I've got to prepare myself for a new culture, a new place, and you consciously think about that. But nobody consciously thinks that there's any preparation needed to come home, because it's home. Well, when I got back from Azerbaijan, it was nine months in a place that really had nothing. It was a broken down, rusty, crumbling place with nothing. And thirty-six hours later I was in southern California. I recall this so vividly: I was in a supermarket, in the produce section, and my jaw dropped. I was speechless – I couldn't count the number of kinds of apples there were. I was walking around the supermarket in shock.

"I visited an aunt and we were walking down a street, and there were these boxes out behind a restaurant – they were throwing out some vegetables. I was looking at these bell peppers – each one had this little blemish on it, and they were throwing them out. Every single one of those vegetables was in far better condition than the best ones I was buying in the market. I couldn't even hear what she was saying, I was stunned. The roads were so smooth. You turn a knob and there's hot water. It's magic, it's really magic. You know that scene in *Cast Away* where Tom Hanks is in that hotel room and he turns that switch on and off? I looked at that and I said, 'I know what that is.' You can't believe you just flip a switch and the room gets lit.

"I'd get home and I really couldn't relate. I was not nice to be around for weeks and months after some missions. I'd get on my motorcycle and take a sleeping bag and a few books and I'd go away for six weeks and learn a little bit of civility in the process. I got back after Somalia and I was just a mean bastard – I hated everything around me. I was not a nice person."

Lorber recalls how the more experienced volunteers tried to prepare him for the re-entry. "When I took the first training course at MSF there was a joke going around called New Fridge Syndrome: You're going to go off on your mission and you're going to come home, you're going to be sitting at the dinner table with your family, and you're going to want to tell every-thing about your mission – what you saw, the corruption, the dead people, the happy things. And your mother's going to look at you and say, 'Hmm, that's wonderful. Did I tell you we got a new refrigerator?'"

It's those reactions from family and friends that are often the hardest for MSFers to deal with. Everyone at the party wants to hear their stories and see their photos – for a few minutes. Soon the listener's eyes have glazed over and he's thinking about the shrimp cocktail that just went by. "One of the things you miss when you come back," says physician Leslie Shanks, "is that you've been working with a group, all of whom are focused on improving the health of the population, improving the situation. And then you come home and nobody cares. Even though when you're away you're missing your family and your friends, it's very difficult to come back because people don't understand – some people don't want to understand, other people can't understand. There's also this sense that it's too much for them to hear. It's difficult to be in this space where you can't share your experiences because of the traumatic effect it's going to have on the listener. And those are the people who *are* interested and want to hear about it. On the other side you've got all these people who can't even identify on a map where you've been to. 'Which continent is that on? Oh, is there a war there?' You've just seen people slaughtered in front of your eyes, and even your being there can't stimulate your acquaintances."

Some returned expats are burning to share their stories and raise awareness in their own countries. But they soon realize that people don't want to be told how lucky they should feel, how minor their own problems are. When they flush the toilet, they don't want to be reminded that some refugee in a faraway land doesn't get that much water in a day. There's a danger, too, of giving people the impression that you think their whole lives are self-indulgent and frivolous. "Reintroducing yourself into life as you knew it before is difficult," says Patrick Lemieux, "because it's a hell of a change, and everything seems insignificant. You're listening to the complaints of your best friends, and you're like, 'Yeah, so?' You hear a telephone ring and it upsets you. You do become almost antisocial in that respect, at least by Western standards. But that wears off. Then you learn to live your next mission less emotionally. My friends tell me, 'Patrick, you've changed. The first time around you were always complaining, telling us we should feel guilty about this or that; you were saying, let's take the bus rather than the taxi. Now you seem more laid back.' And I think that's true. By the third or fourth mission, it's easier to adjust. It's easier for you to accept these inequities. It's easier for you to accept that people only have a passing interest in what you're doing because they can't relate to it. Those that try to follow it and do take the time to look through photos, videos, with whom you've emailed a lot, they have a better idea, but they don't have ..." His voice trails off. "Nonetheless, they show interest in your stories."

Chris Day agrees that the readjustment varies according to your experience and the difficulty of the mission but also relates to what you do when you get back. An MSF colleague offered him a suggestion: "He said, 'Don't go back to what you thought was comfortable and familiar, because if you feel alienated from what's comfortable and familiar to you, you'll have a really hard time. Go do something completely different, completely out of your regular cultural pattern. Go to a tractor pull." Where you don't want to go, says Day, who lives in Charleston, South Carolina, is to a mecca of consumerism. "It was really hard coming back from Sierra Leone. It was awful. I spent a month in New York when I got back, and New York is not the place to be. It's sensory overload. After a month I had stress-induced alopecia – I lost some hair. In New York, you may as well pin twenty-dollar bills on your clothes and walk outside so people can snatch them off of you. A lot of it is financial distress, because in MSF the money sucks.

"After Ivory Coast I had only one bad day. What really kicked it off was I needed to buy a pair of jeans, and I went to the mall in Charleston. That's a bad place to be around Christmas, when you've just come back from Africa. And it was really like, 'Man, I shouldn't be here.' The bad days are when I feel that the things people around me see as significant are quite a lot different from what I've done with my life. People construct their identities around what they consume. And everyone's getting married and buying a house and a car, and I'm not. You start to wonder, 'Am I supposed to be doing that? Am I supposed to be getting mutual funds?' You just start to panic, like, 'Oh my God, I'm doing this wrong. I'm falling behind.' You freak out because you're one step away from homelessness. But that was only a day."

For doctors and nurses returning from the field, there may be an added hurdle of readjusting to their medical practice. In developing countries, it's a daily occurrence to see patients showing up at the health center, after having walked for hours, with diseases so advanced there's no hope of saving them. Then they come home to waiting rooms full of people with runny noses. For some, it's simply not an issue. "I don't find that a problem at all," says one doctor, "because our role as physicians is to deal with what the person feels is the problem. And people's problems expand to fill their lives. So, I'm really sorry, ingrown toenails here are just as big a deal as whatever the Third World problem is. My job is not to judge the severity of people's problems." Another doctor admits that his MSF travels have caused him to question the Western tendency to treat terminal illnesses aggressively, but they haven't affected his day-to-day patient care. "When I see a kid with a sprained ankle, I don't say, 'What the hell are you doing here? If you were in a refugee camp ...' What does that mean? It's totally irrelevant. You have to get over it."

Others find it's not so easy to move between the worlds. "I've been working in the emergency department of a children's hospital for three years now," says Leanne Olson, who lives in Quebec, "and from day one till now it bugs me the way parents will come in with this fast-food mentality toward health care. 'I have ten minutes, could you see my child now and fix him? I have an appointment.' Where do you come by this sense of entitlement and this selfishness? There are really sick kids there, and they don't care. They want their child seen right now. The first year was terrible – I honestly didn't know if

I could stay. It was the first time I had been back working in a hospital after MSF, and then working in the Netherlands with refugees. Coming back here was such a blow. There are still times when I have to bite my tongue so I don't say: 'You know, your health care is some of the best in the world, and it's free. So shut up.' I hated going to work sometimes."

Nurse Carol McCormack had her own difficulties when she returned from Africa to work in a tiny community in northern Canada, just inside the Arctic Circle, where substance abuse is common. "I like to take care of people who haven't done this to themselves, and I really had a problem dealing with the drinking-related stuff – people calling me in the middle of the night, getting yelled at, cursed at. When I got back from Burundi, I had even less of a tolerance for it. I remember having no sympathy for my patients and really having to cover that up, because that could have got me in trouble. I did say it overtly to some patients – I had to watch my mouth. But it faded. I just wanted to take them by the shirt and shake them and say, 'You're so damn lucky. You have a life, you're relatively healthy, you don't risk being shot every day, you can be vaccinated for meningitis.' We had one patient here die from TB. We did everything in our power to x-ray people, give them tests – they were just swamped by medical people. That's one of the top three illnesses in Burundi. They don't know how lucky they are. They abuse themselves, and they abuse each other."

Shortly after settling in, McCormack sent an email to a colleague who was considering writing an article about their Burundi experience:

We had a murder here last Tuesday. First one in five years – not too bad for a community of 850. As I performed

CPR on this man's lifeless body, I was surprised to note how detached I felt. He'd attacked someone and then got stabbed in the chest – both of them were screaming drunk. Later, when we pronounced him dead, I felt no empathy for the man, nor for the family. No sadness. The two nurses I worked with that night were quite freaked out. When they offered us "debriefing and counseling" the next day, I almost laughed. What has happened to empathetic and sensitive Carol? I always feared this would be my reaction when I returned home. My time in Burundi has set a new precedent, a new definition of what matters, what true suffering is. It ain't the man with the bleeding head requiring sutures because he got into a fight – calling me a fucking bitch the whole time. It isn't the person on the phone who has been drinking for six weeks straight and now can't stop vomiting and wants Valium, or the woman who can't stop coughing because she has been smoking since she was twelve. My tolerance for these cases is in the gutter, but I am getting good at pretending that I care.

An article on Burundi – a great idea. You could write about Jeanine, that fourteen-year-old girl who got caught in crossfire in Butaganzwa and received a bullet through her frontal lobe, or the family in the bed next to her who lost their four-month-old in the same fighting. They also couldn't find their two other children. I remember the look on the father's face the day he found them. What about the woman who wailed when her sixteen-year-old daughter died of meningitis in the health center, or the malnourished boy in the feeding center who had been so swollen by malnutrition that his skin was starting to weep and peel off? He died that night. Or the father who asked me to check his little girl with swollen feet. I didn't have time, it was late, so I asked him to come back the next day. Next time we saw him, we heard the little girl had died. "That's how things go," he said.

I remember your comments about first missioners providing that fresh look, new eyes. I am a little sad that I won't have those eyes if I do another mission.

It is snowing and dark now at 3 p.m. Nothing to do but walk the dog and visit friends. It is true, nobody really wants to hear about Burundi. I am talking on the local radio this Tuesday. I will keep it very simple. I would love to tell them how fortunate they are to live in a country with such great access to health care, even if it sucks by Canadian standards.

Even if no one else does, there are always colleagues who understand. "I got back from Nigeria, and that was a brutal mission," says Peter Lorber. "That is really a terrible, screwed-up place – but wonderful at the same time. There was so much on my mind and in my heart. I'm sitting at the table and my family is saying, 'Tell us about Nigeria.' I should have known better, but I couldn't help myself, and I said, 'Well, there are clashes in the north in Kaduna, and they were putting tires around people's heads; and then down in Biafra there's this and that; and over in Lagos, you wouldn't believe what this slum looked like.' And my mother literally sat there and went, 'Wow. Did I tell you we got a new refrigerator?' I swear to God. I couldn't believe it. And I thought, 'Those guys at MSF really know what they're talking about.'"

10 | You Can't Stop a Genocide with Doctors

Stretched out in the TV room of the Médecins Sans Frontières house in Kandahar, Hernan del Valle reflects on the reasons he volunteered with MSF. An Argentine human-rights lawyer with a wicked sense of humor, del Valle has worked with several other aid organizations, including Save the Children and Oxfam, but he says only MSF has the *cojones* "to tell everyone else to fuck off."

That glibness has prompted other aid organizations to label MSF as arrogant, self-righteous troublemakers. Nonetheless, it's part of del Valle's job as humanitarian affairs officer for Afghanistan and Pakistan to try to ensure that other organizations – the UN High Commissioner for Refugees, the two countries' governments, foreign-aid donors – are doing what MSF believes is best for the population, and he speaks out publicly when they're not. It's part of what MSF calls *témoignage*.

The literal meaning of *témoignage* is "witnessing," though it is more often translated as "advocacy." Even that doesn't capture the nuance of the term, so MSFers tend to use the French word regardless of their native tongue. The organization's main role has always been delivering medical aid, but even if advocacy makes up a small fraction of its activities – 5 or 6 percent of its operating costs – it's an important part of its identity. One MSFer puts it this way: "Chimpanzees share ninety-eight percent of our DNA. *Témoignage* is like our two percent – it's what distinguishes us from other NGOs." The idea goes all the way back to Bernard Kouchner and Biafra, though it's not easy to pin down, and MSF admits that it's a source of continuous debate. The criteria for speaking out are fluid; individuals have their own interpretations of when it is appropriate, and prevailing views are different among the sections. Jean-Hervé Bradol, president of MSF-France – where the concept perhaps has the most resonance – says it's misleading to think about delivering medical aid and *témoignage* as two entirely separate actions. "From my point of view, there isn't such a distinction between speaking and acting. I think we permanently speak out, in a way." He's referring to the idea that the mere presence of an international NGO offers some deterrent to injustice.

Speaking out has its price, however, and not only in other organizations' ill will. It also goes against the principle of neutrality, a pillar of humanitarianism, and it puts teams in the field at risk of retaliation. After treating hundreds of brutally raped women and children in Sudan's Darfur region, for example, the Dutch section published a report on the abuse in March 2005. The eight-page document stopped short of blaming Khartoum explicitly, but it described how most of the attackers wore military uniforms and stated that local authorities were tolerating the crimes. The Sudanese government demanded that the organization produce evidence for the claims, and when it wasn't satisfied, it arrested two MSF staffers, Paul Foreman and Vincent Hoedt, and charged them with crimes against the state in late May. The charges were later dropped, but human rights groups report that aid workers in the country have been routinely threatened by Sudanese troops.

The consequences of criticizing a regime are serious enough for expats; for the populations they serve, however, they can be far more dire. While an international team can pull out of a project that becomes dangerous, their local staff has no such luxury. One MSFer remembers an overzealous head of mission he worked with in Colombia, a "stupid cowboy" who talked about going to the media with a list of human rights violations he witnessed. "The local staff turned white and said, 'If you do that they're going to kill my family tomorrow.'"

In extreme cases, where MSF publicly denounces a regime, it must withdraw from the country – as it did in Ethiopia in 1985, and more recently in North Korea in 1998. The population it had been serving, however imperfectly, may then be left with no health care, which is why denunciation is a last resort, an exasperated admission that all other avenues have failed. Drawing the world's attention to human rights violations is not the core business of MSF, as it is for groups like Amnesty International or Human Rights Watch. But when a suffering population needs more than health care and no one else is around to say that, or when medical aid is being abused, MSF will stretch its mandate. "During the famine in North Korea," says Rony Brauman, "we realized that everything we were bringing – whether medical services or high-protein food – was being used by the North Korean regime to strengthen itself. It was a resource for the perpetrators, and not a resource for the victims." Rather than be manipulated, MSF chose to withdraw its teams from the country and publicly expose the situation. "The idea is that it's a cost in terms of public image to endure documented criticism by an NGO. So we can establish a kind of balance of power — we don't have weapons, we don't have anything we can threaten the country with. But we can blur its image; we can weaken it."

Brauman also feels that MSF is justified in speaking out when it is the only witness to massive crimes against civilians. That happened in Angola in 2002, when the organization was the first NGO to enter some areas after the war ended. "We came across vast groups of the population in an appalling state — starvation, extreme weakness due to forced labor, slavery, rapes, terrible things. Those people had been used as slaves by both the government forces and the guerrilla forces. We were the only witnesses of this, and we decided we had to report on it, because if we didn't say anything nobody would, and we couldn't keep this to ourselves."

Then there is the pragmatic element of MSF's advocacy work, the one that Hernan del Valle put into practice when he went to bat for displaced Afghans. Here, again, MSF is criticized for appointing itself the guardian of the population's interest and assuming it always knows what's best. And here, too, del Valle plays MSF's trump card: the independence that comes from raising most of its own funds. "In this job you have the luxury of saying, 'I am advocating for the people.' And who can go against that? You can actually go to a meeting and say, 'We're not asking for more water for this camp because we want more money from UNHCR. It's because people need to drink.'" He says other NGOs will grudgingly admit they wished they had the same freedom to speak up, but they worry about losing contracts from the UN or government agencies. "They will tell you off the record, 'We agree with what you're saying, we think that's the right principle, but our salaries come from there.'" That's why journalist David Rieff, who has written critically about how aid agencies can be co-opted by donor interests, has said that MSF "is both envied and resented by other groups. It is, in an important sense, the conscience of the humanitarian world."

In March 2002, UNHCR and the Afghan and Pakistani governments began the enormous effort of helping hundreds of thousands of Afghan refugees go home. By August 2003, some 2.3 million had returned from Pakistan and Iran, with another 10,000 or so following every week. On the surface, it sounded like a good-news story. But, according to MSF, not all of them were moving willingly. "MSF has been against the repatriation in Afghanistan, and very vocal, because we think it is premature," says del Valle. UNHCR has a formal mandate to uphold international refugee law – which includes a refugee's right not to be repatriated against his will – and if MSF believes it is failing in that responsibility, it will scream and shout.

Pakistan had already accepted more refugees than it felt it could handle, and it closed its border at Chaman in February 2002. Some 25,000 Afghans were trapped in a no-man's-land that came to be called the Waiting Area. "A big and somewhat ridiculous debate about their status began," del Valle says. "The discussion revolved around a patch of desert, a total space less than three hundred meters south or north of the line dividing the two countries." Put simply, the people in the Waiting Area needed food, water and medical care, and MSF says no one wanted to provide it – not Afghanistan, not Pakistan and not

UNHCR. "All the actors interpreted the situation in a way in which they could get away without providing assistance."

For their part, UNHCR and both governments argued – fairly, even MSF would concede – that the improvised Waiting Area had none of the services of an official refugee camp. Water had to be brought in by truck, sanitation was inadequate and the whole area was dangerous, as coalition forces clashed with the resurgent Taliban in nearby towns. In May 2003, the refugees in the Waiting Area were given a choice: return to their homes, move to Mohammed Kheil (a camp deeper inside Pakistan), or relocate to the newly erected Zhare Dasht camp on the Afghan side of the border, where they would no longer be classed as refugees but as internally displaced people. After a mass exodus in July, almost 11,000 ended up in Zhare Dasht, while some 7,800 agreed to move to Mohammed Kheil. There they received the food and other aid that comes with official refugee status.

The relocation addressed one of MSF's concerns, but by this time the Waiting Area had been occupied for 15 months and people were just beginning to adapt to life there. Because the settlement was so close to the towns of Chaman and Spin Boldak, del Valle says, some of the inhabitants had even found work. "Ironically, when people finally had developed survival strategies, adapted to the place, built their mud houses, and got some daily labor in the bazaar, they were informed that they had to leave the area without delay and move again into other temporary settlements – not a durable solution, but just another relocation." The population, MSF argued, was manipulated. "There were push factors that undermined their ability to choose freely – to get food you had to register to move. Having said that, when we saw the decision to move them was irreversible, MSF decided to concentrate on damage control. We concentrated our advocacy on *how* the relocation was going to be carried out and tried to get the best deal for the refugees, since we could not do anything else at that point. Staying behind – as most of them wanted to do – was no longer an option."

"It was on 8 December 2000, at 8:30 in the evening, that we were attacked by government soldiers who took us for rebels, but they were mainly interested in stealing." The words are read in musical tones by a young Congolese man in front of a small audience in a downtown Toronto auditorium. He's narrating a passage from a book of testimonies collected by MSF teams in the Democratic Republic of Congo. This is the story of André, a father of three in Katanga. "They grabbed my bicycle, extorted medicines from my nephew, a member of the Red Cross, and took the belt from my little brother's trousers. The soldiers hit me. It is painful to admit that our own soldiers beat us, but it's true. That's what happens."

Even if the people in the audience that evening were acquainted with the ongoing war in DRC, chances are most had never heard the first-hand stories of individuals living through it. Congo is home to some of the organization's biggest medical projects, and, according to one MSFer in the region, it is "among the greatest humanitarian disasters of our time." Yet every year, the country shows up on MSF's list of the world's most underreported humanitarian stories. Even when African conflicts make the news in the West, the numbers are simply too large to register – millions displaced, hundreds of thousands killed. Sometimes *témoignage* is less about changing policies than about simply giving voice to suffering individuals like André, to dispel the idea that people in DRC and other war-torn countries have become inured to violence and don't suffer as acutely as people in the West. "That's complete and utter bull-shit," says an MSF doctor who has done three missions in the country. "The difference is that they don't give up."

MSF's advocacy is based on first-hand observation, not reports from other groups, and is backed up by solid evidence. The organization, in fact, has developed expertise at tracking disease outbreaks, doing nutritional surveys and collecting epidemiological data in emergencies. In 1987, MSF created Epicentre, a Paris-based consulting organization that offers these services to other NGOs. No one questions the value of this information, but within MSF there are those who feel this type of *témoignage* is overly technical and gets away from a fundamental principle of humanitarianism – that it is a compassionate response to suffering and doesn't need to be justified by science. "In modern life, and this goes way beyond MSF, there's a tendency to overvalue things that can be quantified," says Richard Bedell, who has been an adviser on medical ethics for MSF-Holland. "There's an idea in the modern rational mind that if you can put a number to it, it's somehow harder and more reproducible, and more real than anything that you can't put a number to. It's an unexamined assumption that what's quantifiable and calculable is probably superior."

If the French have historically been the passionate voice of *le mouvement*, Holland has been the section most likely to lean in the overly pragmatic direction Bedell warns about. "I feel nowadays that the Dutch section is closer to the core ideas of MSF than it was back when I started to work at headquarters in

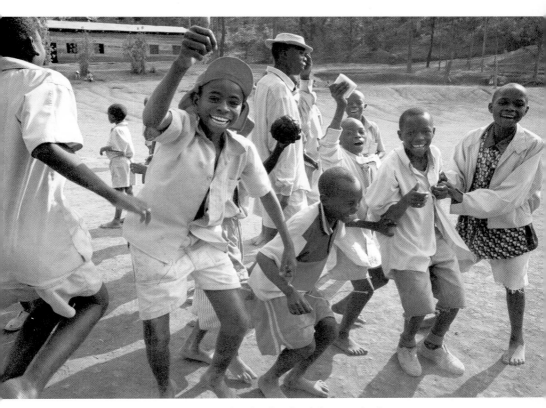

Rwandan children at Ishwa Island School celebrate winning an MSF-sponsored drama competition, in which the students performed plays about the importance of clean water.

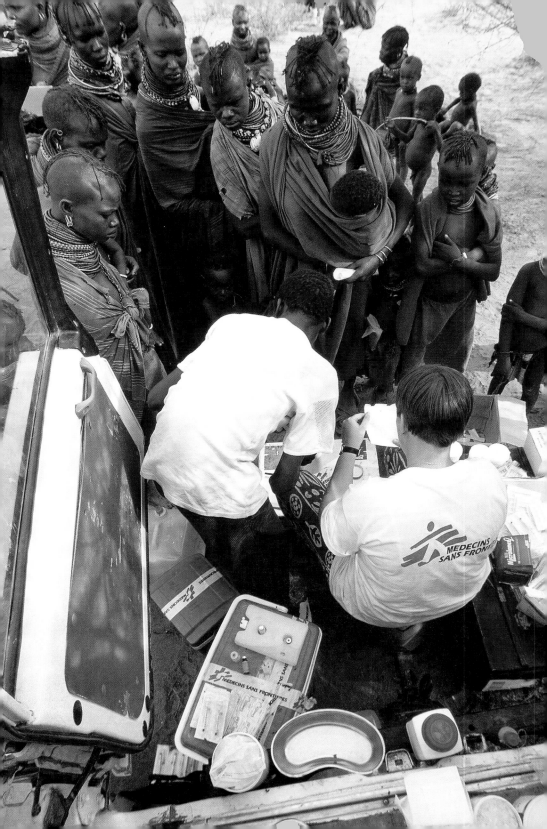

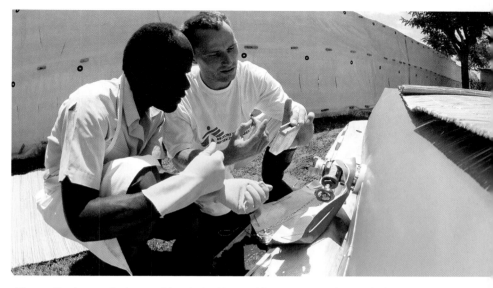

Above: During a cholera epidemic in Mozambique, MSF engineers help deliver clean water to a hospital in Maputo. As well as working in acute emergencies, "watsans" bring water and sanitation to isolated villages.

Opposite: Nomads in the Turkana region of northern Kenya receive basic health care from an MSF mobile clinic, usually a pair of Land Cruisers stocked with medicines and a small team of expats and national staff.

An MSF doctor examines the chest x-ray of an AIDS patient who is also suffering from tuberculosis, one of the deadly opportunistic diseases that strike people with HIV.

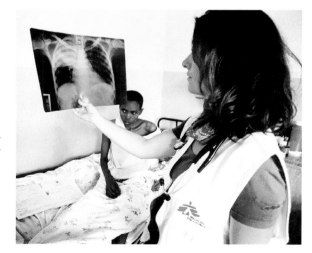

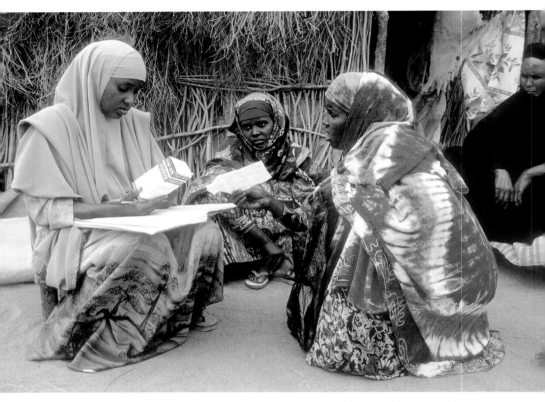

A nurse visits refugee women during an MSF psychosocial program in the Dadaab camps in Kenya, near the Somali border. Tens of thousands of people have been living in the camps for more than a decade.

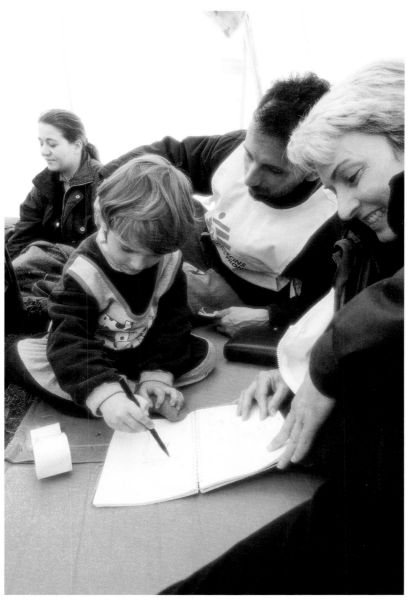

While some within the organization would prefer to focus on purely medical activities, MSF has also used drama and art therapy. In this 1999 program, Kosovar children are drawing pictures about their experiences.

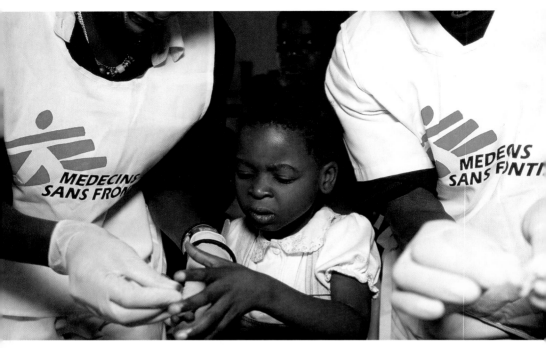

Above: An Angolan child gives a blood sample to MSF staff as part of a case-finding mission. On these trips, medical teams travel from village to village to test people for signs of infectious diseases.

Below: A national staff member registers a patient in Busia, a region of Kenya on the border with Uganda, where MSF has run an AIDS program since 2000. Up to a third of Busia's population is believed to be HIV-positive.

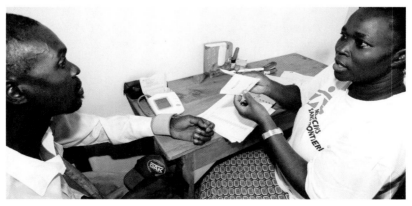

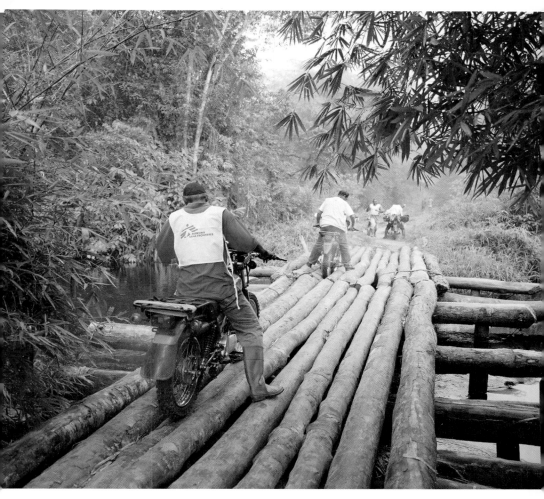

Motorbikes are the only way in to the Djolu region of the Democratic Republic of Congo. To get to patients in remote areas, medical teams will also travel by bicycle, river boat or on foot.

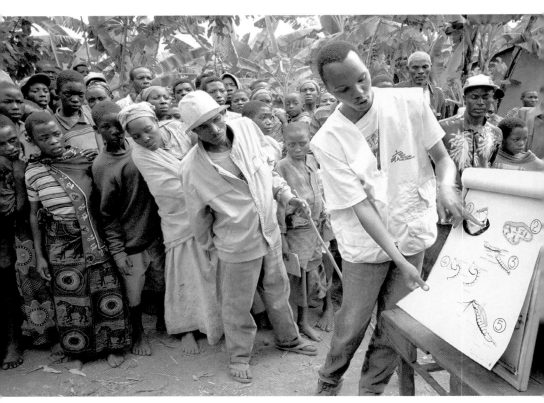

As part of an anti-malaria program in Burundi, an MSF technician explains the life cycle of the mosquito to a group of villagers. While prevention is crucial, MSF is also lobbying for better treatment of the disease with artemisinin-based drugs.

1996," he says, "when I felt that they were drifting perilously away from some core issues in the charter. I felt they were heading toward a certain kind of public-health approach. There are some really good ideas in public health and a lot of good methods, but it missed a lot of what's ethically important at MSF, such as the regard for the specific individual. That kind of thing, which is preserved within the classic MSF view, can get lost if you overemphasize the public-health perspective."

Being on the ground, interacting directly with patients and their families, is part of that classic MSF view, and it challenges medical volunteers to put their own value judgments on hold. Bedell recalls running a project in Taliban-controlled Afghanistan and meeting a man who refused to let male caregivers treat his wife. "It's important to remind yourself that, except in the most bizarre, extreme situation, a man does not want to harm his wife. A man does not want to see his wife die, even in Afghanistan. He simply doesn't see the choice. That's what we can't forget. We can't forget to respect people, even if we don't understand. Because trying to change people from a stance other than respect is hopeless. To coerce, to ridicule, will never work. I don't think we do this very well. There is some general exposure to the phenomenon of cultural difference during the preparatory course that most people do before their first field mission, but even with our best efforts, one would find situations that one didn't expect. So what you need to do is equip people with a certain attitude for learning, a certain readiness to observe, listen and learn."

Whether expat humanitarian workers can ever show true solidarity with the people to whom they deliver aid is questionable. "I'm less convinced than many people in MSF," says Fiona Terry, research director at Fondation Médecins Sans

Frontières, the organization's think tank in Paris. "I don't know if the presence of someone with an MSF T-shirt is going to make me feel any better. I'm rather uncomfortable with this notion of solidarity. I think in some respects in MSF it's become too much of a slogan. I mean, what do we really mean by it? We don't live by their side, we go back to our comfortable houses at night, we drive in our nice four-wheel drives, we have all the modern conveniences of email, we can talk with our friends and family. Can we really say we're in solidarity with them? It sounds nice, it makes us feel better, but it might be naïve to think that victims in the field feel this."

Some relief NGOs employ local staff almost exclusively in the field, with expats acting only as managers working in the capitals. MSF has made a conscious decision not to follow that model. "From the very beginning we wanted to promote the relationship between societies," says Jean-Marie Kindermans of MSF-Belgium. "MSF is to help people, but it's also to have people meeting each other from different societies, to increase tolerance, to increase understanding. It's a richness to put together people from different cultures, and it's a richness that the people coming from Europe, meeting volunteers in other countries, come back and speak to their own society." As the organization has grown, it has struggled to hold on to this ideal of proximity. In 2002, for example, MSF reported that its operational costs rose 19 percent over the previous three years, while its number of field positions increased only 5 percent. "We are getting more and more office-heavy," wrote Morten Rostrup, international president at the time; "the weight of the field in relative terms is reduced." In an internal paper, Rostrup related how he had recently made a visit to the field, where he was picked up by a black BMW and driven to the

gated MSF compound, complete with satellite TV, two refrigerators and laptops with satellite modems. None of the expats
on the team did any direct consultations with patients.

> When I asked if this really was necessary, I got the
> answer that this was the least MSF could do when they
> "sacrificed" themselves to the benefit of the locals ... I
> wondered whether some of the volunteers, despite
> being there physically, were really *mentally* in the field
> ... What kind of relationship did we actually have to the
> people that were living there, the people we assisted
> with health care? What kind of relationship do we
> expect if we fence ourselves away from the local popu-
> lation, if we drive in our big white Land Cruisers, if we
> only have social contact with other expats, if we never
> treat the patients ourselves? What does the MSF slogan
> "proximity" really mean?

Martin Girard sums it up this way: "We've got more people
behind computers and fewer people sitting around the fire
with the poor bastard in South Sudan, trying to understand
the guy." For Girard, humanitarian action is intensely personal, and even if he and the South Sudanese never fully
understand one another, there's value in just being there
around that fire. "You get involved in this kind of organization
because of your feeling of human solidarity, that's the bottom
line. Do you feel any solidarity with an African who is in shit
up to his eyeballs, or not? It's a very simple question, and I
answer yes, one hundred percent. I'm motivated to stand side
by side with these guys and say, 'Some of the people where I
come from benefit from your situation, but I don't agree with

that, and I'm here to show you that we're not all the same.' The locals witness your efforts, and they respect that. But when you get to a village they're not on their knees going, 'Thank you, thank you, white man from MSF, we're so happy to see you.' MSF vehicles have gotten rocks thrown at them, spears and arrows, because they didn't handle the situation well, or they fucked up in the field.

"We're not anthropologists, but when you're in the bush in South Sudan and you're dealing with the Dinka and the Nuer, you're on Mars. There's absolutely nothing that links these people to your way of life. These are hunters and cattle herders and nomads, and they have a thousand-year history. But you strive to understand their suffering, what they have been through. Your understanding of it will always be imperfect. You think you, with your white ass, are going to understand after three months in the field? But they say, 'Wow, you didn't forget about us.' This is where the solidarity comes in, because you leave a rich country, or a nice livelihood, and you jump in the shit up to your shoulders with them for nine hundred bucks a month."

Chris Day says that when MSF rolls into town, the receptiveness of the population varies widely. "In Kashmir, we were the only NGO there, and people don't have a wide range of experience with expatriates coming into their villages. It was mixed – Kashmir has a highly educated population, and you have quite a few people who will say, 'Go home to your country and tell them what's going on here,' and others will come flat out and say, 'You're just an instrument of the American government. Go away with your cultural imperialism.' In African countries like Liberia and Sierra Leone, where NGOs have been coming and going for over a decade, humanitarian aid, NGOs, and expatriates just become part of how society functions, because we're providing substitutions for a lot of services that don't exist. They become part of how people survive.

"I can totally understand why some people think it's self-indulgent to talk about solidarity. It *is* self-indulgent. MSF was founded very much to give white doctors from Europe an opportunity to experience a Third World country – very French. And that loosely translates into solidarity now."

People in crisis, however, are often buoyed by knowing the world hasn't forgotten about them. "I am absolutely convinced that it matters to people," says Richard Bedell. "Sometimes they even realize that it matters more than the technical assistance." He knows volunteers in Kosovo and Chechnya who have been told as much by the population. "That sense that the world knows they're there, and that they're suffering, is tremendously important. We don't want to *just* make symbolic acts, but we shouldn't underestimate the importance of them either, in terms of motivating people to help themselves. We're not giving assistance to a bunch of people sitting around passively with their hands open. It's an interactive thing, and if we can give them some hope, they're able to interact with us much more successfully. That's part of what we're giving."

"I'm not trying to suggest that the solidarity that MSF shows is somehow better than what another organization would show," says physician Michael Schull. "But it is true that some organizations don't utilize expatriates as much. Refugees may be poor and powerless, but they're rarely stupid. They recognize how the world works, and the fact that many of our expatriates come from countries that are relatively powerful politically."

Schull saw this when he worked among Burmese refugees in Bangladesh. The Bangladeshi government was bent on sending the refugees back against their will, even though it violated international law. Many UNHCR officials in the camp were Bangladeshis who did not speak the refugees' language, and people questioned the validity of their interviews. "There was concern that the translations were not being done accurately, that the refugees were being made to appear that they wanted to go home when they didn't. And we used to get notes thrown to us by refugees as our cars were coming in or leaving the camp. They didn't want to be seen passing us information, but they were saying, 'We're being sent home against our will; please get this message out to the world.'"

If humanitarian agencies ever felt that their presence among people in crisis was an uncomplicated act of goodness, that notion died in Rwanda.

On April 6, 1994, extremist Hutus, Rwanda's ethnic majority, began their meticulous slaughter of some 800,000 Tutsis and moderate Hutus. Urged on by propaganda that spilled from radios, the killers began house-by-house searches for Tutsi "cockroaches" and systematically cut them down with machetes. That spring, the three largest MSF sections – France, Belgium and Holland – all had teams on the ground, mostly working with people displaced by the ongoing conflict in both Rwanda and neighboring countries. But while some of these teams had been in the region for several years and had seen countless atrocities, nothing would prepare them for what they were about to witness.

Just two days after the massacres began, MSF-France decided to evacuate its team from a camp in southeastern Rwanda.

Thirty expats and about 50 locals, mostly Tutsis, climbed into a dozen vehicles and headed for the Burundi border, where they had arranged to meet with MSFers based on the other side. When they arrived at customs, however, they were told the Rwandans would not be allowed to leave the country. After hours of negotiation, darkness began to fall and the officials announced that the border would close at 6 p.m. The expats were forced to make the decision to leave their staff behind as they crossed into Burundi. In his end-of-mission report, a French logistician described the chilling scene:

> At 5:15 p.m., "A" [an MSF expat] was still negotiating, but only for four Tutsi women who were certain to be killed. The customs officers still refused point blank. "A" started to shout out loud, which created consider- able tension and led to a temporary break in the nego- tiations. Then the coordinators of each camp made their decision ... Emotional scenes followed. I said good-bye to my driver, who had been with me for sev- eral months, and to others who I liked a lot, but I felt I had done all I could to try and get them to come with us. Other expats burst into tears at the sight of them leaving. "A," depressed by his failure, went to find the [expat] coordinators and informed them bluntly that they would have the death of thirty Rwandans on their conscience. He was still convinced we could have got them through, that nothing could happen to a group of thirty expats overnight at the border ...
>
> There was a rift in the group between the majority, who had wanted to go through without the staff, and the others who thought that we should have continued

to negotiate, that we had let forty people go to their deaths. In Bujumbura, during sessions organised by two headquarters staff who had come to help us "air our dirty laundry," all the animosity came out.

The coordinators' difficult decision to go ahead without the Rwandan staff had been the right one. It was out of the question that we should spend the night with those soldiers who had no commanding officer and were drunk as well. Moreover, MSF cannot infringe the laws of the host country. The Rwandan staff continued to work in the camps, but we heard that seventeen of them were killed, and, no doubt, the rest met with the same fate.

Then on April 22 and 23, in the southern city of Butare, 150 Tutsi patients in the hospital were hacked to death in front of the MSF medical staff. When the Hutu soldiers grabbed a Rwandan nurse – seven months pregnant and a close friend of the expat team – one of the Belgian doctors stepped in: "They came to take Sabine and I intervened physically and said, 'Leave Sabine alone. Sabine has nothing to do with this ... and besides, she is a Hutu.' The captain who was responsible for the different teams looked at me very carefully, and then he opened his pocket and took out a piece of paper, and on this piece of paper there was a list of names, typed. And Sabine's name was on it. He looked at the paper and he looked at me and said, 'Yes, you are right. Sabine is a Hutu. But her husband is a Tutsi. And his baby is going to be a Tutsi.' I suddenly realized the cruel reality that in Rwanda the baby follows the paternal line. So Sabine was killed and so was the baby."

By the middle of April, MSF began to discuss whether it

should make an official public declaration about what was happening in Rwanda, despite the attendant problems of singling out the Hutus. For aid workers on the ground, being perceived as anything other than neutral could be a death sentence. As it was, some MSF doctors in Rwanda defected to the ICRC, feeling that the Red Cross's discretion would offer them more safety. MSF, for its part, decided that discretion was no longer an option and, on May 13, the Paris office went public with the news that almost a hundred of their Rwandan staff had been murdered. The desire to speak out, while not unanimous, was particularly fervent in France, because the government of François Mitterrand was an ally of the Hutu regime. On May 18, MSF-France spent 70,000 francs to publish an open letter to Mitterrand in *Le Monde*: "Mr. President, the international community, and France in particular, must accept its political responsibilities and put a stop to the massacres." After the letter appeared, Jean-Hervé Bradol said in a television interview that "the French state knows these people [the Hutu regime] only too well, since it has provided them with equipment." Mitterrand's advisers later requested a meeting with MSF, where Bradol was told, "You must know that the president took your TV interview rather badly. That wasn't very bright of you."

As the weeks progressed and the UN continued to dither, MSF-France made an unprecedented decision. On June 7, the board agreed to call for an armed intervention to stop the genocide. In its 23-year history of working in the most brutal wars, MSF had never before taken this step, nor has it done so since. Some argued that it was inappropriate for a humanitarian organization to call for a military offensive under any circumstances. They wondered, too, whether the French government, already considering an intervention, would exploit MSF's position for its own political gain. The majority, however, believed that using force to stop the killings was the only ethical response, and one entirely sanctioned by international law. (The 1948 Convention on the Prevention and Punishment of the Crime of Genocide, to which Rwanda is a signatory, not only permits but *requires* other states to intervene to halt a genocide.) On June 17, when MSF-France held a press conference to present its case, it used the unforgettable slogan *On n'arrete pas un génocide avec des médecins.* You can't stop a genocide with doctors.

Between July and September, the French army carried out Operation Turquoise to establish safe havens in Rwanda. Although the intervention and its motives were highly controversial, it slowed the exodus of refugees and probably saved thousands of Tutsi lives. But the problems were far from over for Rwanda and for MSF. In Tanzania, Zaire (as the DRC was then called) and Burundi, huge numbers of Rwandan refugees had already gathered. Immediately after the killing began in April, the Tutsi-dominated Rwandan Patriotic Front (RPF) launched a counterattack, and by the end of the month a quarter of a million Hutus had fled across the Tanzanian border. In those early days of the refugee crisis, aid workers could honestly claim they believed that the Hutus were simply fleeing the advance of the RPF. By early June, though, they could see that Hutu military leaders were orchestrating the exodus from Rwanda, dragging civilians along with them. Their plan was carefully laid out in documents later uncovered in the camps: once they crossed the borders into the waiting arms of aid agencies, these mass murderers would extort international relief and use it to finance their regime. They would use the protection of the camps to rest, regroup and plot their return

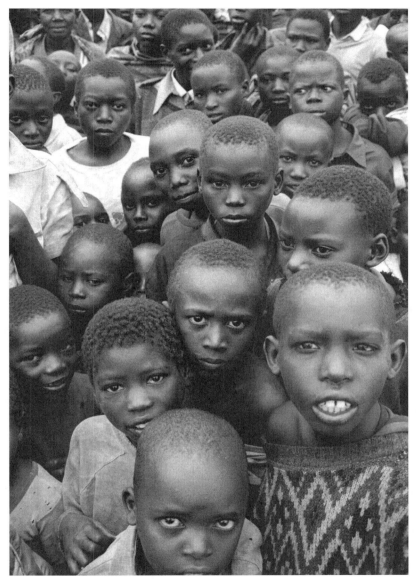

A year after the Rwandan genocide, refugee children arrive at a camp on the Burundi–Tanzania border. The killing of some 800,000 Tutsis and politically moderate Hutus in 1994, and the subsequent exodus from Rwanda, forced MSF to confront the dilemmas of providing aid.

to Rwanda to finish the genocide they had started. The aid groups, unwittingly, played right into their hands.

In July, as many as 800,000 more Rwandan refugees – again, mostly Hutus coerced by their leaders – crossed into Goma, Zaire, in just four days. Almost immediately, there were massive cholera and dysentery outbreaks. By July 28, MSF reported 14,000 deaths in Goma, and the ultimate toll may have been 50,000. The Belgian and Dutch sections moved to intervene, and Leslie Shanks was among the doctors who flew to Zaire that summer with MSF-Holland. "I remember very clearly thinking on the plane that this would really be a test of my humanitarian principles. In June and July we still didn't have a very good picture of what had happened during the genocide, but I knew that *génocidaires* were in the camp where I was going – people who had perpetrated an incredible massacre – and I was going to save them. But when it comes right down to it, I'm a medical person, and if someone's sick it doesn't matter what they've done before or what they're going to do. If they're sick, my job is to treat them, not to make judgments about them. Nobody deserves to die from a simple thing like cholera, which is so easy to treat."

Once the cholera was under control, however, some people in MSF began to question whether they could still justify that logic. In late August, a third wave of refugees – up to 400,000 – settled in Bukavu, Zaire. Now some 2 million Hutus were stationed just outside their home country. "As for us," said a senior MSFer, "we're just running along behind." Fiona Terry, then MSF-France's head of mission in Tanzania, would later write: "It is not unusual for aid to have unavoidable side effects. But in the case of the Rwandan camps, it was nothing *but* the aid which was sustaining the viability of the old regime." On top of all this, aid workers were receiving death threats if they acted against the wishes of the Hutu leaders. MSF began to mutter about pulling out and publicly denouncing the situation. An agency with limited funds can't help every suffering population, but can it refuse to give aid on moral grounds? What about the Hutu civilians in the camp who were not killers? Would MSF abandon the women and children in its programs to die while it took a principled stand? If MSF was aware that its aid was being manipulated, did that make it an accomplice? These were just a few of the questions the teams hotly debated on October 14, when they met in the Rwandan capital of Kigali to discuss what to do next.

During the Kigali meeting, representatives from France, Holland and Belgium tried to arrive at a consensus, but it proved impossible. To varying degrees, the Dutch and the Belgians argued that it would be better to stay in the camps in the short term and deliver health care, while at the same time documenting the abuse and lobbying governments for improvements. (When these improvements never happened, the Belgian and Dutch sections decided in 1995 to withdraw as well.) MSF-France, in contrast, unilaterally announced on October 28 that it was withdrawing from Tanzania and Zaire within a month. This decision upset many people in the other sections and even some within MSF-France – they felt the office had ignored the teams in the field. Any time headquarters proposes evacuating a team, emotions run high in the field, where expats have developed a bond with their local staff and their patients. In Rwanda, these emotions had been magnified tenfold. "I remember being proudly told in my initial briefings that MSF is an association where everyone has an equal voice," an angry Fiona Terry wrote in a fax to Paris after learning that her team would have to leave Tanzania. "At the time I realized that was an exaggeration but I never realized the extent of this farce until today."

Many other relief organizations debated the situation in the Rwandan refugee camps, but in the end the US-based International Rescue Committee was the only other major group to pull out, citing reasons similar to those of MSF-France. As David Rieff points out, their position was like that of a conscientious objector:

> It was a complicated gesture, at once principled and hollow. For while it was important that NGOs take such a stand ... there were other relief groups already poised to take the place of those who withdrew ... The real question, and it was one that, fortunately for them, neither IRC nor MSF had to face, was whether they would have withdrawn in a situation that was analogous politically, but in which they were the only aid groups on the scene.

Rwanda was a watershed for Médecins Sans Frontières and the entire humanitarian community. Aid had been abused before, agencies manipulated and refugee camps used as sanctuaries by exiled military regimes. But never before had the stakes been so high and the role of aid agencies so integral to the strategy of the perpetrators. "It pushed all of us in MSF to reflect deeply on what humanitarian action represents," Fiona Terry writes, "and at what point it loses its sense and becomes a technical function in the service of evil."

More than a decade later, that reflection continues. As the 10th anniversary of the genocide approached in the spring of

2004, MSF's international office decided there would be no *témoignage* campaign to commemorate the event. For the doctors who could not stop a genocide, the wounds opened in Rwanda still have not healed.

The horror of Rwanda, and the impossible situation it created for Médecins Sans Frontières and other agencies, was the most dramatic example of the limits of humanitarian action. But it was not the first one, nor the last. From Biafra to the ongoing conflict in Iraq, more than three decades of intervention have muddied whatever moral clarity may have once existed in the aid community. Only the hopelessly naive are blind to the dilemmas of providing assistance – and yet, at the same time, only the hopelessly cynical have given up on the idea. As James Orbinski explained in his Nobel lecture, "Today we struggle as an imperfect movement, but strong in thousands of volunteers and national staff, and with millions of donors who support, both financially and morally, the project that is MSF."

Indeed, even as so much has been called into question, MSF not only survives but has arguably become the most respected aid agency in the world. Its leaders have shown a remarkable ability to adapt, to stay relevant and to lead by example, and the organization's influence goes well beyond its own health clinics and feeding centers. "While it is impossible to overstate the value of what MSF has achieved in the past," David Rieff wrote after the Nobel Prize, "the group's next great accomplishment may be to rescue and redefine the ideal of humanitarianism itself."

The attacks of September 11, 2001, and the subsequent wars in Afghanistan and Iraq were opportunities to do just that, and MSF quickly learned that the task wouldn't be easy. That October, many longtime donors in North America were outraged when MSF argued that the US military's food drops for Afghan civilians were both cynical and dangerous. The organization knew about the risk from experience – its doctors have treated patients who were injured after mistaking cluster bombs for relief packages or who entered mined areas to collect food. Some of the provisions may also have ended up in the hands of combatants, and in any case they were hopelessly inadequate to address the hunger. Above all, however, the military was, as an MSF press release declared, "shooting with one hand and delivering medicines with the other."

Since that time, the co-optation of humanitarian action has become the single greatest threat to groups like MSF. Humanitarian NGOs must remain third parties in a conflict, not allies of one side or the other, and they must be perceived as neutral. But by dropping aid packages as well as bombs, the US-led coalition firmly positioned itself as part of a team that included humanitarians. "More than ever, governments and intergovernmental organizations must work in partnership with NGOs if compelling problems are to be effectively addressed," Secretary of State Colin Powell said on October 26, 2001. "As I speak, just as surely as our diplomats and military, American NGOs are out there serving and sacrificing on the front lines of freedom." Even the NGOs themselves, many of which are funded by the United States and other Western governments, allowed the line to be blurred.

In the circumstances, it wasn't surprising. During those emotional weeks after September 11, when North Americans felt the world had changed overnight, people wanted something they could be sure of. They wanted to believe that humanitarian groups were the good guys, our partners in the fight against the evil terrorists. "The first media call I had to deal with showed how successful the propaganda of the food drops was," says David Morley, executive director of MSF-Canada at the time. "The reporter said to me, 'When I was having my Thanksgiving dinner, I felt so thankful that we were dropping food as well as bombs. Now, are you telling me I was wrong to feel like that?'"

That's exactly what MSF was saying, though few people wanted to hear it. Undaunted, MSF stuck its neck out and argued that it wasn't on anyone's side, except that of the sick and hungry. "We need to maintain a real distance from political and military actors, even though they may be from our society," says Nicolas de Torrente, executive director of MSF-USA. "Culturally, historically, politically, of course, we are closer to the US government than to the most radical Islamic groups. But we need to really believe in our principles rather than just pay lip service to them." Impartiality during war is a fundamental tenet of humanitarianism, but it's tough to sell that amid the rhetoric of "if you're not with us, you're against us." MSF knew it was correct, however, and by the time American and British forces invaded Iraq in March 2003, even its harshest critics admitted as much. "Now, if you talk about the US using humanitarian aid to try to win over hearts and minds in a propaganda effort in Iraq, everyone says, 'Of course,'" de Torrente said later that year. "It's everywhere, it's in the newspapers, it's not a problem. But right after September 11 it was just about impossible to make that point."

In the weeks leading up to Operation Shock and Awe in Iraq, MSF again showed its leadership. While some American NGOs refused to take funding from the US Agency for International Development because they recognized the conflict of interest, others made no such choice and became, in Rony Brauman's words, "subcontractors to a belligerent party." At the opposite end of the spectrum, some European aid organizations, under pressure from the general public to speak out against the impending war, actively opposed a military strike on Iraq because of the human suffering it would cause. MSF responded by asking how these NGOs knew that a US invasion would be worse than Saddam Hussein's dictatorship. They argued – if not uniquely in the aid community, at least more forcefully than anyone else – that it is not for humanitarians to ask who is right in a war, but only who needs help. Peace is not their business, even if it is their desire. Individuals within MSF admit they sometimes find this frustrating, but they recognize it can be no other way. In the end, that is perhaps MSF's greatest strength.

Humanitarians can face one of two pitfalls: they can ignore the possible dangers of delivering aid and proceed blindly with a stubborn single-mindedness, or they can throw up their hands and argue that no aid is better than aid that might do harm. With equal parts brains, balls and heart, MSF has managed to avoid both traps. Its doctors and nurses accept the limits of the aid they deliver, and they constantly question their own work. Yet they do not dither in a crisis – on the contrary, the group gets its people on the ground, delivering medical aid as quickly as any other NGO. MSF may wring its hands, but it does not bind them.

Médecins Sans Frontières cannot save the world, and it long ago stopped pretending it could. "Many of us would like to do more," says David Morley. "We would like to see a more just world, but we have to focus on what we can do. And what we can do is something simple, small and profound."

That's more than a drop in the ocean; it's a lifeboat. It may not stop the ship from going down, but it saves lives and, more important, it promises hope.

"Ours Is Not a Contented Action"

Excerpts from Dr. James Orbinski's Nobel Peace Prize acceptance speech

On December 10, 1999, Dr. James Orbinski, then international president of Médecins Sans Frontières, delivered the traditional lecture as the organization accepted the Nobel Peace Prize.

Given the formality of the occasion, he might have been forgiven for offering only bromides and ingratiating platitudes, but that wouldn't have been MSF's style. Instead, Orbinski immediately drew attention to one of the worst humanitarian crises in the world at that time: "The people of Chechnya – and the people of Grozny – today and for more than three months, are enduring indiscriminate bombing by the Russian army."

It was a provocative opener, and much of what followed had equal power. Here is a shortened version of the acceptance speech.

Let me say immediately that the extraordinary distinction that the Nobel Committee has given Médecins Sans Frontières is one that we accept with sincere gratitude, but also a profound discomfort in knowing that the dignity of the excluded is assaulted daily. These are the forgotten populations in danger, like the street children who struggle each grinding hour to live off the waste of those who are *included* in the social and economic order. These too are the illegal refugees that we work with in Europe, denied political status, and afraid to seek health care, lest this contact leads to their expulsion.

Our action is to help people in situations of crisis. And ours is not a contented action. Bringing medical aid to people in distress is an attempt to defend them against what is aggressive to them as human beings. Humanitarian action is more than simple generosity, simple charity. It aims to build spaces of normalcy in the midst of what is abnormal. More than offering material assistance, we aim to enable individuals to regain their rights and dignity as human beings. As an independent volunteer association, we are committed to bringing direct medical aid to people in need. But we act not in a vacuum, and we speak not into the wind, but with a clear intent to assist, to provoke change, or to reveal injustice. Our action and our voice is an act of indignation, a refusal to accept an active or passive assault on the other.

The honor you give us today could so easily go to so many organizations, or worthy individuals, who struggle in their own society. But clearly, you have made a choice to recognize MSF. We began formally in 1971 as a group of French doctors and journalists who decided to make themselves available to assist. This meant sometimes a rejection of the practices of states that directly assault the dignity of people. Silence has long been confused with neutrality, and has been presented as a necessary condition for humanitarian action. From its beginning, MSF was created in opposition to this assumption.

We are not sure that words can always save lives, but we know that silence can certainly kill. Over our 28 years we have been – and are today – firmly and irrevocably committed to this ethic of refusal. This is the proud genesis of our identity, and today we struggle as an imperfect movement, but strong in thousands of volunteers and national staff, and with millions of donors who support both financially and morally, the project that is MSF.

Humanitarianism occurs where the political has failed or is in crisis. We act not to assume political responsibility, but firstly to relieve the inhuman suffering of failure. The act must be free of political influence, and the political must recognize its responsibility to ensure that the humanitarian can exist. Humanitarian action requires a framework in which to act.

In conflict, this framework is international humanitarian law. It establishes rights for victims and humanitarian organizations and fixes the responsibility of states to ensure respect of these rights and to sanction their violation as war crimes. Today this framework is clearly dysfunctional. Access to victims of conflict is often refused. Humanitarian assistance is even used as a tool of war by belligerents. And more seriously, we are seeing the militarization of humanitarian action by the international community.

In this dysfunction, we will speak out to push the political to assume its inescapable responsibility. Humanitarianism is not a tool to end war or to create peace. It is a citizens' response to political failure. It is an immediate, short-term act that cannot erase the long-term necessity of political responsibility.

And ours is an ethic of refusal. It will not allow any moral political failure or injustice to be sanitized or cleansed of its meaning. The 1992 crimes against humanity in Bosnia-

Herzegovina. The 1994 genocide in Rwanda. The 1997 massacres in Zaire. The 1999 actual attacks on civilians in Chechnya. These cannot be masked by terms like "complex humanitarian emergency" or "internal security Crisis." Or by any other such euphemism – as though they are some random, politically undetermined event. Language is determinant. It frames the problem and defines response, rights, and therefore responsibilities. It defines whether a medical or humanitarian response is adequate. And it defines whether a political response is inadequate. No one calls a rape a complex gynecologic emergency. A rape is a rape, just as a genocide is a genocide. And both are a crime. For MSF, this is the humanitarian act: to seek to relieve suffering, to seek to restore autonomy, to witness to the truth of injustice, and to insist on political responsibility.

The work that MSF chooses does not occur in a vacuum, but in a social order that both includes and excludes, that both affirms and denies, and that both protects and attacks. Our daily work is a struggle, and it is intensely medical, and it is intensely personal. MSF is not a formal institution, and with any luck at all, it never will be. It is a civil society organization, and today civil society has a new global role, a new informal legitimacy that is rooted in its action and in its support from public opinion. It is also rooted in the maturity of its intent, in for example the human rights, the environmental and the humanitarian movements, and of course, the movement for equitable trade. Conflict and violence are not the only subjects of concern. We, as members of civil society, will maintain our role and our power if we remain lucid in our intent and independence.

Today, a growing injustice confronts us. More than ninety percent of all death and suffering from infectious diseases occurs in the developing world. Some of the reasons that people die from diseases like AIDS, TB, sleeping sickness and other tropical diseases is that life-saving essential medicines are either too expensive, are not available because they are not seen as financially viable, or because there is virtually no new research and development for priority tropical diseases. This market failure is our next challenge. The challenge, however, is not ours alone. It is also for governments, international government institutions, the pharmaceutical industry and other NGOs to confront this injustice. What we as a civil society movement demand is change, not charity.

We affirm the independence of the humanitarian from the political, but this is not to polarize the good NGO against bad governments, or the virtue of civil society against the vice of political power. Such a polemic is false and dangerous. As with slavery and welfare rights, history has shown that humanitarian preoccupations born in civil society have gained influence until they reach the political agenda. But these convergences should not mask the distinctions that exist between the political and the humanitarian. Humanitarian action takes place in the short term, for limited groups and for limited objectives. This is at the same time both its strength and its limitation. The political can only be conceived in the long term, which itself is the movement of societies. Humanitarian action is by definition universal, or it is not. Humanitarian responsibility has no frontiers. Wherever in the world there is manifest distress, the humanitarian by vocation must respond. By contrast, the political knows borders, and where crisis occurs, political response will vary because historical relations, balance of power, and the interests of one or the other must be considered. The time and space of the humanitarian are not those of the political. These vary in opposing ways, and this is another way to locate the founding principles of humanitarian action: the refusal of all forms of problem solving through sacrifice of the weak and vulnerable. No victim can be intentionally discriminated against, or neglected to the advantage of another. One life today cannot be measured by its value tomorrow: and the relief of suffering *here*, cannot legitimize the abandoning of relief *over there*. The limitation of means naturally must mean the making of choice, but the context and the constraints of action do not alter the fundamentals of this humanitarian vision. It is a vision that by definition must ignore political choices.

Humanitarian action comes with limitations. It cannot be a substitute for political action. In Rwanda, early in the genocide, MSF spoke out to the world to demand that genocide be stopped by the use of force. And so did the Red Cross. It was, however, a cry that met with institutional paralysis; with acquiescence to self-interest, and with a denial of political responsibility to stop a crime that was *never again* to go unchallenged. The genocide was over before the UN Operation Turquoise was launched.

There are limits to humanitarianism. No doctor can stop a genocide. No humanitarian can stop ethnic cleansing, just as no humanitarian can make war. And no humanitarian can make peace. These are political responsibilities, not humanitarian imperatives. Let me say this very clearly: the humanitarian act is the most apolitical of all acts, but if actions and its morality are taken seriously, it has the most profound of political implications. And the fight against impunity is one of these implications.

This is exactly what has been affirmed with the creation of the international criminal courts for both the Former Yugoslavia and Rwanda. It is also what has been affirmed with the adoption of statutes for an International Criminal Court. These are significant steps. But today, on the 51st anniversary of the Universal Declaration of Human Rights, the court does not yet exist, and the principles have only been ratified by three states in the last year. At this rate it will take 20 years before the court comes into being. Must we wait this long? Whatever the political costs of creating justice for states, MSF can and will testify that the human costs of impunity are impossible to bear.

Yes, humanitarian action has limits. It also has responsibility. It is not only about rules of right conduct and technical performance. It is at first an ethic framed in a morality. The moral intention of the humanitarian act must be confronted with its actual result. And it is here where any form of moral neutrality about what is good must be rejected. The result can be the use of the humanitarian in 1985 to support forced migration in Ethiopia, or the use in 1996 of the humanitarian to support a genocidal regime in the refugee camps of Goma. Abstention is sometimes necessary so that the humanitarian is not used against a population in crisis. More recently, in North Korea, we were the first independent humanitarian organization to gain access in 1995. However, we chose to leave in the fall of 1998. Why? Because we came to the conclusion that our assistance could not be given freely and independent of political influence from the state authorities. We found that the most vulnerable were likely to remain so, as food aid is used to support a system that in the first instance creates vulnerability and starvation among millions. Our humanitarian action must be given independently, with a freedom to assess, to deliver and to monitor assistance so that the most vulnerable are assisted first. Aid must not mask the causes of suffering, and it cannot be simply an internal or foreign policy tool that creates rather than counters human suffering. If this is the case, we must confront the dilemma and consider abstention as the least of bad options. As MSF, we constantly call into question the limits and ambiguities of humanitarian action – particularly when it submits in silence to the interests of states and armed forces.

Independent humanitarianism is a daily struggle to assist and protect. In the vast majority of our projects it is played out away from the media spotlight, and away from the attention of the politically powerful. It is lived most deeply, most intimately in the daily grind of forgotten war and forgotten crisis. Numerous peoples of Africa literally agonize in a continent rich in natural resources and culture. Hundreds of thousands of our contemporaries are forced to leave their lands and their family to search for work, food, to educate their children and to stay alive. Men and women risk their lives to embark on clandestine journeys only to end up in a hellish immigration detention center, or barely surviving on the periphery of our so called civilized world.

Our volunteers and staff live and work among people whose dignity is violated every day. These volunteers choose freely to use their liberty to make the world a more bearable place. Despite grand debates on world order, the act of humanitarianism comes down to one thing: individual human beings reaching out to their counterparts who find themselves in the most difficult circumstances. One bandage at a time, one suture at a time, one vaccination at a time. And, uniquely for Médecins Sans Frontières, working in around 80 countries, over 20 of which are in conflict, telling the world what they have seen. All this in the hope that the cycles of violence and destruction will not continue endlessly.

As we accept this extraordinary honor, we want again to thank the Nobel Committee for its affirmation of the right to humanitarian assistance around the globe. For its affirmation of the road MSF has chosen to take: to remain outspoken, passionate and deeply committed to its core principles of volunteerism, impartiality, and its belief that every person deserves both medical assistance and the recognition of his or her humanity. We would like to take this opportunity to state our deepest appreciation to the volunteers and national staff who have made these ambitious ideals a concrete reality, and who have, we believe, brought some peace to the world that has experienced such immense suffering and who are the living reality of MSF.

Author's Note

Médecins Sans Frontières is an extraordinary organization in many ways, not least in the way its volunteers generously shared their stories for this book. Many related difficult memories with candor; I hope they feel their trust was well placed.

I am grateful to the MSF-Holland teams who welcomed me into their homes and compounds in the field, especially James Knox, Maria-Elena Ordoñez, Martha Anderson, Mónica Rodríguez, Carla Peruzzo, Ya-Ching Lin, Peter de Bakker, Sebastiaõ Vemba, Mattias Ohlson, Patrick Lemieux, Bertien van Gijssel, Hernan del Valle, Kathleen Bochsler, David Croft, Gerhard Schmid, Benjamin Ugbe, Maarten Van Herk, Tracy Cabrié and Michel Plouffe.

MSF-Canada was unfailingly supportive. Special thanks to Tommi Laulajainen and David Morley for believing in the project from the beginning, Madeleine Favre for arranging my travel, and Carol Devine for her encouragement. Above all, *grosses bises* to Isabelle Jeanson for her enduring friendship on three continents.

At MSF-USA in New York, thank you to Nicolas de Torrente, Kris Torgeson and Kevin Phelan.

Physicians Christa Hook and Richard Bedell patiently and articulately explained technical subjects and corrected my misunderstandings. I bear full responsibility for any that may remain in the text.

Of the many people outside MSF who shared their insights, I am particularly indebted to two of them. Renée Fox, professor emerita of sociology at the University of Pennsylvania, read a portion of the manuscript and offered wise suggestions and random acts of encouragement when I needed them most. Amanda Allan of the University of Melbourne, a researcher in the psychosocial effects of humanitarian aid work, was inexplicably generous in sharing her findings with me.

Thank you to Lionel Koffler, Michael Worek and Brad Wilson at Firefly Books for an unparalleled opportunity; to Rosemary Shipton, my superlative editor, who supplied the clear-headed direction I needed to turn the first draft into a final manuscript; and to Maria DeCambra for her intrepid photo research.

My deepest appreciation goes to Wendy, for putting up with the physical and emotional absence this book required and for welcoming me home when the work was done.

Notes on Sources

Between 2002 and 2004, I conducted almost a hundred interviews with MSFers, as well as academics and objective outsiders. I spent several weeks visiting teams in Angola, Afghanistan and Pakistan, as well as the MSF offices in Amsterdam, Brussels, New York, Montreal and Toronto. These interviews provided the bulk of the material in these pages.

The notes that follow are not comprehensive but include the sources I have quoted in the text, those that provided the most helpful background, and those that are readily available to readers interested in learning more about MSF and humanitarian aid.

The aid community benefits from a number of excellent news services available on the web, including Reuters AlertNet (www.alertnet.org) and ReliefWeb (www.reliefweb.int), both of which I consulted extensively.

MSF reports, press releases and internal documents were, of course, invaluable research material, though I have listed only the most important here. Many are available on MSF websites, including www.msf.org, www.doctorswithoutborders.org, and www.msf.ca.

Introduction: Fixing Up the Humans

David Rieff's comments: *A Bed for the Night: Humanitarianism in Crisis* (New York: Simon & Schuster, 2002), 83.

The golden age of humanitarianism: Tony Vaux, *The Selfish Altruist: Relief Work in Famine and War* (London: Earthscan, 2001), 43ff.

Chapter 1: Under the Angolan Sun

Angola from the 1970s to the 1990s: Ryszard Kapuscinski, *Another Day of Life* (New York: Vintage, 2001); Karl Maier, *Angola: Promises and Lies* (London: Serif, 1996); see also the Human Rights Watch report, *Angola Unravels: The Rise and Fall of the Lusaka Peace Process* (1999).

MSF activities in Angola from 2000 onward are explained in a series of reports, including *Angola: Behind the Façade of "Normalization"* (November 9, 2000), *Angola: After the War Abandonment* (August 2002), and *Angola: Sacrifice of a People* (October 2002); see also Zoe Eisenstein, "Angola Refugees Begin Slow Road Home," Reuters, February 21, 2003.

Disagreement with United Nations: MSF press release, "Thousands of Angolans Left to Starve" (June 11, 2002); UN Office for the Coordination of Humanitarian Affairs press release, "OCHA Angola's Response to MSF Statement" (June 11, 2002); see also the editorial "Beyond Trading Insults in International Humanitarian Aid," *The Lancet*, June 22, 2002, 2,125.

Chapter 2: Biafra and the Bumblebee

Bernard Kouchner biographical details: Michael Ignatieff, *Empire Lite* (Toronto: Penguin Canada, 2003); "Charlemagne: Bernard Kouchner, Controversial Proconsul for Kosovo," *The Economist* (US), July 19, 1999, 48; Carol Devine et al., *Human Rights: The Essential Reference* (Phoenix: Oryx Press, 1999); John Hanc, "Healing the World," *Runner's World*, December 1993, 36.

Influence of the Paris milieu on Kouchner: Renée C. Fox, "Medical Humanitarianism and Human Rights: Reflections on Doctors Without Borders and Doctors of the World," in Jonathan Mann et al., eds., *Health and Human Rights: A Reader* (New York: Routledge, 1999), 419.

Neither of the two most comprehensive sources on the early history of Médecins Sans Frontières is available in English. Olivier Weber's *French Doctors: Les 25 ans d'épopée des hommes et des femmes qui ont inventé la médicine humanitaire* (Paris: Robert Laffont, 1995) covers the two and a half decades that followed the Biafran war. I am indebted to Geneviève Séguin for translating portions of this book. Dorthe Ravn's *Læger Uden Grænser* (Frederiksberg, Denmark: Bogfabrikken Fakta, 1998) was also invaluable, with thanks to Kurt Dahlgaard for providing an unpublished English translation by René Bühlmann. See also Rony Brauman, "The Médecins Sans Frontières Experience," in Kevin Cahill, ed., *A Framework for Survival* (New York: Basic Books, 1993), and Patrick Aeberhard, "A Historical Survey of Humanitarian Action," *Health and Human Rights* 2, 1 (1996): 31–44.

Kouchner's personal reflections on Biafra: "From Doctors Without Borders to Patients Without Borders," lecture delivered at the Harvard School of Public Health, March 6, 2003. See also Alvin Powell, "Kouchner Calls for Global Health Care," *Harvard University Gazette*, March 13, 2003.

History of humanitarian intervention: David Rieff, *A Bed for the Night: Humanitarianism in Crisis* (New York: Simon & Schuster, 2002); Hans Köchler, "Humanitarian Intervention in the Context of Modern Power Politics" (Vienna: International Progress Organization, 2001); Francis A. Boyle, "Humanitarian Intervention: A Joke and a Fraud," Doctor Irma M. Parhad Lecture, University of Calgary, 2001; Philippe Guillot, "France, Peacekeeping and Humanitarian Intervention," *International Peacekeeping*, spring 1994, 31.

Bernard Kouchner and the development of humanitarian intervention: Tim Allen and David Styan, "The Right to Interfere? Bernard Kouchner and the New Humanitarianism," *Journal of International Development*, August 2000, 825–42; Mary Kaldor, "A Decade of Humanitarian Intervention: The Role of Global Civil Society," in *Global Civil Society Yearbook 2001*, Helmut Anheier et al., eds. (London: London School of Economics, 2001); Hugo Slim, "Military Intervention to Protect Human Rights: The Humanitarian Agency Perspective" (International Council on Human Rights Policy, 2001); Olivier Corten, "Humanitarian Intervention: A Controversial Right," UNESCO *Courier*, July/August 1999, 57–59. I am grateful to Tim Allen of the Development Studies Institute at the London School of Economics for help in providing historical context and perspective.

Rony Brauman's comments on MSF's intervention in Afghanistan and Cambodia: Médecins Sans Frontières, *World in Crisis: The Politics of Survival at the End of the 20th Century* (New York: Routledge, 1997).

Jacques de Milliano's journal of Sudan: Anke de Haan, Edith Lute and Roderick Bender, *Médecins Sans Frontières: 10 Years Emergency Aid Worldwide* (Amsterdam: MSF-Holland, 1995).

Harry and Marijke in Sudan: Peter Dalglish, *The Courage of Children* (Toronto: HarperCollins, 1998), 270–80.

French citizens' desire to work for MSF: Ronald Koven, "Crisis Alert: Volunteer Medics Heal the World," *The World & I*, July 1989.

Chapter 3: We Don't Need Another Hero

The most articulate personal account of life inside MSF is Leanne Olson's *A Cruel Paradise: Journals of an International Relief Worker* (Toronto: Insomniac Press, 1999).

Motivations of MSF volunteers: Elliott Leyton and Greg Locke, *Touched by Fire: Doctors Without Borders in a Third World Crisis* (Toronto: McClelland & Stewart, 1998).

Recruiting and training: Michael J. VanRooyen, "Emerging Issues and Future Needs in Humanitarian Assistance," *Prehospital and Disaster Medicine*, October–December 2001, 216–22; Rachel T. Moresky et al., "Preparing International Relief Workers for Health Care in the Field: An Evaluation of Organizational Practices," *Prehospital and Disaster Medicine*, October–December 2001, 257–62.

Michael Maren's comments: *Might Magazine*, March/April 1997, quoted at www.netnomad.com/might.html.

Chapter 4: Doc in a Hard Place

Dominique Larrey and the history of emergency medicine: M.K.H. Crumplin, "Surgery in the Napoleonic Wars," *Journal of the Royal College of Surgeons of Edinburgh*, June 2002, 566–78; Miguel A. Faria Jr., "Dominique-Jean Larrey: Napoleon's Surgeon from Egypt to Waterloo," *Journal of the Medical Association of Georgia*, September 1990, 693–95; Robert L. Pearce, "War and Medicine in the Nineteenth Century," *ADF Health (Journal of the Australian Defence Health Service)*, September

2002; Moshe Feinsod, "The Surgeon and the Emperor: A Humanitarian on the Battlefield," in Aryeh Shmuelevitz, ed., *Napoleon and the French in Egypt and the Holy Land, 1798–1801* (Istanbul: Isis Press, 1999).

Chapter 5: In the Yellow Desert

Background on Kandahar and southeastern Afghanistan: Christina Lamb, *The Sewing Circles of Herat* (Toronto: HarperCollins, 2002); Eliza Griswold, "Where the Taliban Roam," *Harper's*, September 2003, 57–65; Daniel Bergner, "Where the Enemy Is Everywhere and Nowhere," *New York Times Magazine*, July 20, 2003; Phil Zabriskie, "Undefeated: On the Afghanistan–Pakistan Border, the Taliban Are Regrouping, Bent on Spreading Terror," *Time* (Asia edition), July 21, 2003; United Nations High Commissioner for Refugees, particularly the report "Return to Afghanistan" at www.unhcr.ch.

Medical needs of displaced people: Médecins Sans Frontières, *Refugee Health: An Approach to Emergency Situations* (London: Macmillan, 1997); Rony Brauman, "Refugee Camps, Population Transfers, and NGOs," in Jonathan Moore, ed., *Hard Choices: Moral Dilemmas in Humanitarian Intervention* (Lanham, Md.: Rowman & Littlefield, 1998).

Siege of Mir Wais hospital: Ellen Knickmeyer, "U.S., Afghan Forces Kill al-Qaida Holdouts," Associated Press, January 28, 2002; Michael Ware, "Dead Men Talking," *Time*, February 2, 2002.

Attacks on humanitarian workers in Afghanistan: Mercy Corps, "A Lesson from Afghanistan: The Price of Unfinished Business," ReliefWeb, April 29, 2003; Françoise Chipaux, "The Taliban Are Back in Southeast Afghanistan," *Le Monde*, April 5, 2003; Todd Pitman, "Two Afghan Red Crescent Workers Killed; UNHCR Attacked," Associated Press, August 14, 2003; Sayed Salahuddin, "Four Aid Workers Killed in Afghan Ambush," Reuters AlertNet, September 10, 2003.

Slaying of five workers in Badghis: MSF press release, "MSF Shocked by Death of 5 Staff in Afghanistan," June 3, 2004; Stephen Graham, "Agency Halts Its Afghan Operation," Associated Press, June 4, 2004; Marianne Stigset, "Humanitarian Ideals Die with Aid Workers in Afghanistan," *Daily Star* (Lebanon), June 4, 2004; interview with Samuel Hauentein of MSF-Holland, *As It Happens*, CBC Radio (Toronto), June 3, 2004.

Chapter 6: Ugly Realities

Nobel committee press release and presentation speech: Nobel e-Museum, www.nobel.se/peace/laureates/1999/press.html; www.nobel.se/peace/laureates/1999/presentation-speech.html.

Joelle Tanguy's comments: "Controversies Around Humanitarian Interventions and the Authority to Intervene," speech delivered at the University of California, Berkeley, November 6, 1999.

David Rieff's comment on Kosovo: *A Bed for the Night: Humanitarianism in Crisis* (New York: Simon & Schuster, 2002), 198; italics in original.

Attack in Ethiopia: MSF press release, "MSF Team Attacked in Ethiopia: One Person Killed, One Badly Injured," February 8, 2000.

Fundraising and activities after the South Asian tsunami: MSF internal report, "Six Months After the Asia Tsunami Disaster," June 21, 2005.

Mental health programs: Kaz de Jong, Nathan Ford and Rolf Kleber, "Mental Health Care for Refugees from Kosovo: The Experience of Médecins Sans Frontières," *The Lancet*, May 8, 1999, 1,616–17; Kaz de Jong et al., "Psychological Trauma of the Civil War in Sri Lanka," *The Lancet*, April 27, 2002, 1517; Richard F. Mollica, "Mental Health and Psychological Effects of Mass Violence," in Jennifer Leaning, Susan M. Briggs and Lincoln Chen, eds., *Humanitarian Crises: The Medical and Public Health Response* (Cambridge, Mass.: Harvard University Press, 1999).

Chapter 7: How the Other Half Dies

James Orbinski's experience in Rwanda: Sarah Scott, "Dr. Orbinsky's [sic] Long Road Home," *National Post* (Toronto), January 4, 2003.

MSF's Nobel acceptance speech: Nobel e-Museum, www.nobel.se/peace/laureates/1999/msf-lecture.html; see also Michael Schull, "MSF, the Nobel Peace Prize, and the Canadian Connection," *Peace Magazine*, winter 2000.

Background on malaria: Fiammetta Rocca, *The Miraculous Fever-Tree* (New York: HarperCollins, 2003); MSF Access to Essential Medicines (www.accessmed-msf.org); Medicines for Malaria Venture (www.mmv.org); Wellcome Trust (www.wellcome.ac.uk); UN Roll Back

Malaria (www.rbm.who.int; mosquito.who.int); World Health Organization (www.who.int); UNICEF (www.childinfo.org).

MSF and artemisinin-based combination therapy: MSF report, ACT *Now to Get Malaria Treatment That Works in Africa* (April 2003).

Dispute in Ethiopia: Ethiopian Federal Ministry of Health press release, "The Malarial Situation in Africa," December 23, 2003; also reports from IPS-Inter Press Service (www.ips.org) and UN Integrated Regional Information Networks (www.irinnews.com).

Background on HIV/AIDS: Tony Barnett and Alan Whiteside, *AIDS in the Twenty-First Century* (Hampshire, UK, and New York: Palgrave Macmillan, 2002); Elizabeth Reid, "A Future, If One Is Still Alive: The Challenge of the HIV Epidemic," in Jonathan Moore, ed., *Hard Choices: Moral Dilemmas in Humanitarian Intervention* (Lanham, Md.: Rowman & Littlefield, 1998); UNAIDS (www.unaids.org).

MSF and antiretroviral treatment: MSF report, *AIDS: The Urgency to Treat* (December 2002); Richard Bedell, "The Introduction of Antiretroviral Therapy in Resource-Poor Settings: Some Ethical Reflections," lecture delivered in Toronto, December 2002; UNAIDS fact sheet, "Access to HIV Treatment and Care," December 2003.

Patent laws and generic drugs: Daryl Lindsey, "The AIDS-Drug Warrior," Salon.com, July 18, 2001; MSF report, *Fatal Imbalance: The Crisis in Research and Development for Drugs for Neglected Diseases* (September 2001); MSF report, *Drug Patents Under the Spotlight* (May 2003); World Trade Organization (www.wto.int).

Anthrax and its effect on the generic-drugs issue: Mike Goodwin, "Prescription Panic: How the Anthrax Scare Challenged Drug Patents," *ReasonOnline*, February 2002; Gardiner Harris, "Bayer's Cipro Will Be Profitable, Even on Discount Deal with U.S.," *Wall Street Journal*, October 26, 2001; V. Sridhar, "Perilous Patent," *Frontline* (India) 18, 24 (November 24–December 7, 2001); Kavaljit Singh, "Anthrax, Drug Transnationals, and TRIPs," *Foreign Policy in Focus*, April 29, 2002.

Canada's potential for leadership on access to generic drugs: James Orbinski, "Access to Medicines and Global Health: Will Canada Lead or Flounder?" *Canadian Medical Association Journal*, January 20, 2004, 224; David Morley, "We Led on AIDS. Why Hang Back Now?" *Globe and Mail*, October 24, 2003, MSF press release, "Bill C-9: How Canada Failed the International Community," April 29, 2004.

Chapter 8: Best Performance in a Supporting Role

Non-medical roles in humanitarian organizations: Carol Bergman, ed., *Another Day in Paradise: International Humanitarian Workers Tell Their Stories* (Maryknoll, NY: Orbis, 2003).

Chapter 9: New Fridge Syndrome

For a complete account of the Fred Cuny case, see the PBS documentary *The Lost American*; www.pbs.org/wgbh/pages/frontline/ shows/cuny.

Delivering medical assistance in Chechnya: Khassan Baiev, *The Oath: A Surgeon Under Fire* (New York: Walker and Company, 2003).

Deaths of aid workers: Dennis King, "Paying the Ultimate Price: An Analysis of Aid-worker Fatalities," *Humanitarian Exchange*, August 5, 2002; Mani Sheik et al., "Deaths Among Humanitarian Workers," *British Medical Journal*, July 15, 2000, 166–68; Francisco Rey Marcos, "When the Red Cross Is the Target," Reuters AlertNet, November 18, 2003; Genevieve Butler, "Afghan Promises Held Ransom by Violence," Reuters AlertNet, December 12, 2003.

Arjan Erkel abduction: Quote from NRC *Handelsblad* in MSF-Switzerland report, "Arjan Erkel: Hostage in the Russian Federation since August 12, 2002," August 12, 2003; Marie Jégo, "MSF accuse des officiels russes de maintenir en otage un de ses volontaires," *Le Monde*, March 10, 2004; Oksana Yablokova, "Mystery Shrouds Erkel's Release," *The Moscow Times*, April 13, 2004; Simon Ostrovsky, "Light is Shed on Erkel's Release," *The Moscow Times*, April 15, 2004; Netherlands Ministry of Foreign Affairs press release, "Déclaration du ministère néerlandais des Affaires étrangères concernant la libération d'Arjan Erkel," May 28, 2004; Natalie Nougayrède, "Les Pays-Bas ont versé une rançon pour la libération d'Arjan Erkel, otage dans le Caucase russe," *Le Monde*, May 29, 2004; Natalie Nougayrède and Jean-Pierre Stroobants, "La polémique monte entre le gouvernement néerlandais et MSF," *Le Monde*, May 30, 2004; interview with Rowan Gillies, *As it Happens*, CBC Radio (Toronto), June 15, 2004.

Psychological toll of aid work: Piet van Gelder and Reinoud van den Berkhof, "Psychosocial Care for Humanitarian Aid Workers: The Médecins Sans Frontières Holland Experience," in Yael Danieli, ed., *Sharing the Front Line and the Back Hills* (New York: Baywood, 2002);

Ruth Barron, "Psychological Trauma and Relief Workers," in Jennifer Leaning, Susan M. Briggs and Lincoln Chen, eds., *Humanitarian Crises: The Medical and Public Health Response* (Cambridge, Mass.: Harvard University Press, 1999).

Rob Gordon, "The Stress of Humanitarian Work," an in-progress paper edited by Amanda Allan and Colleen McFarlane, presented at the Australian NGO Psychosocial Forum, Melbourne, November 2003.

Colin Powell's remarks: US Department of State, "Remarks to the National Foreign Policy Conference for Leaders of Nongovernmental Organizations," delivered in Washington, DC, October 26, 2001.

Tony Blair's remarks quoted in Francisco Rey Marcos, "When the Red Cross Is the Target," Reuters AlertNet, November 18, 2003.

Chapter 10: Doctors Can't Stop a Genocide

MSFers arrested in Sudan: MSF-Holland report, "The Crushing Burden of Rape: Sexual Violence in Darfur," March 8, 2005; Human Rights Watch, "Darfur: Arrest War Criminals, Not Aid Workers," May 31, 2005.

David Rieff on MSF's place among aid agencies: *A Bed for the Night: Humanitarianism in Crisis* (New York: Simon & Schuster, 2002), 83, 187.

Afghan refugees and IDPs: UN Integrated Regional Information Networks (IRIN) report, "Afghanistan: Focus on Chaman Border Crisis," May 7, 2002; IRIN report, "Afghanistan: Special Report on Displaced People in the South," July 21, 2003; UNHCR report, "More than 2.3 Million Returnees since 2001," Afghanistan Humanitarian Update No. 68, August 15, 2003; IRIN press release, "Pakistan: Waiting Area Refugees Subjected to Negative Policies, Says MSF," August 27, 2003; UNCHR press release, "Afghan, Pakistani Governments Agree to Gradually Close Border Camps," August 28, 2003; UNCHR report, "UNHCR's Operation in Afghanistan: Donor Update on Afghanistan," September 8, 2003.

Stories from Democratic Republic of Congo: *Silence On Meurt: Témoignages* (Paris: L'Harmattan, 2002), English excerpts published as *Quiet, We Are Dying* (Toronto: MSF, 2003).

Increasing technical nature of humanitarian aid: David W. Robertson, Richard Bedell et al., "What Kind of Evidence Do We Need to Justify Humanitarian Medical Aid?" *The Lancet*, July 27, 2002, 330–33.

MSF's activity and communications during the Rwanda genocide and its aftermath are meticulously recorded in two internal documents, *Genocide of Rwandan Tutsis, 1994*, and *Rwandan Refugee Camps in Zaire and Tanzania, 1994–1995*, part of the series "Case Studies: Médecins Sans Frontières Speaks Out."

Documents revealing Hutu plans to exploit international aid: Fiona Terry, *Condemned to Repeat? The Paradox of Humanitarian Action* (Ithaca and London: Cornell University Press, 2002), 156.

Cholera and dysentery in Goma, Operation Turquoise and other background on Rwanda: William Shawcross, *Deliver Us from Evil: Peacekeepers, Warlords and a World of Endless Conflict* (New York: Simon & Schuster, 2000).

How aid sustained the Hutu regime in Rwanda: Fiona Terry, *Condemned to Repeat?* 196; long-term effects on MSF, 2. Terry devotes an entire chapter to the situation in the Zairean camps.

David Rieff on the decision to withdraw from Rwanda: *A Bed for the Night*, 187.

James Orbinski's Nobel acceptance speech: Nobel e-Museum, www.nobel.se/peace/laureates/1999/lecture.html.

David Rieff's comments after Nobel Peace Prize: "Good Doctors: Humanitarianism at Century's End," *New Republic*, November 8, 1999, 23.

Criticism of Afghan food drops: MSF press release, "MSF Refuses Notion of Coalition Between Humanitarian Aid and Military," October 6, 2001.

Colin Powell's remarks: US Department of State, "Remarks to the National Foreign Policy Conference for Leaders of Nongovernmental Organizations," delivered in Washington, DC, October 26, 2001.

David Morley's comments: "Humanitarianism in the 21st Century," lecture delivered at the University of Toronto, February 11, 2003.

Aid organizations in Iraq: Rony Brauman and Pierre Salignon, "Iraq: In Search of a Humanitarian Crisis," in Fabrice Weissman, ed., *In the Shadow of "Just Wars": Violence, Politics and Humanitarian Action* (Ithaca and London: Cornell University Press, 2004) 271; see also Jack Epstein, "Charities at Odds with Pentagon: Many Turn Down Work in Iraq Because of U.S. Restrictions," *San Francisco Chronicle*, June 14, 2003.

Potential paralysis in aid organizations: Mary B. Anderson, "You Save My Life Today, But for What Tomorrow? Some Moral Dilemmas of Humanitarian Aid," in Jonathan Moore, ed., *Hard Choices: Moral Dilemmas in Humanitarian Intervention* (Lanham, Md.: Rowman & Littlefield, 1998).

Glossary

ACT: artemisinin-based combination therapy

ARV: antiretroviral

DRC: Democratic Republic of Congo

ECHO: European Commission's Humanitarian Aid Office

EU: European Union

ICRC: International Committee of the Red Cross

IDP: internally displaced person

IRC: International Rescue Committee

MPLA: Popular Movement for the Liberation of Angola

MSF: Médecins Sans Frontières

NGO: non-governmental organization

PC: project coordinator

SFC: supplementary feeding center

SP: sulfadoxine-pyrimethamine

TB: tuberculosis

TFC: therapeutic feeding center

UN: United Nations

UNHCR: United Nations High Commissioner for Refugees

UNICEF: United Nations Children's Fund

UNITA: National Union for the Total Independence of Angola

WHO: World Health Organization

WTO: World Trade Organization

Index

Captions and photographs appear on pages in *italic* type.

Photo Credits

Front Cover, top Hans-Jürgen Burkard, **bottom** Gilles Saussier; **6-7** Abbas/Magnum Photos; **18-19** Dan Bortolotti; **33** MSF; **34** Francesco Zizola/Magnum Photos; **35 top** John Vink/Magnum Photos, **bottom** AP Photo/Ben Curtis; **36** AP Photo/ Ben Curtis; **37** Liba Taylor/Panos Pictures; **38 top** Juan Carlos Tomasi, **bottom** © Noel Quidu/Gamma/PONOPRESSE; **39** © Gilbert Liz/CORBIS SYGMA/MAGMA; **40** Hans-Jürgen Burkard; **47** MSF; **50** MSF; **53** Pascal Deloche; **62** La Poste, France; **90, 95** Wei Cheng; **106** John Vink/Magnum Photos; **110, 112** Dan Bortolotti; **115** Tim Dirven/Panos Pictures; **132** Lloyd Cederstrand; **137** Francesco Zizola/ Magnum Photos; **138 top** Marco Van Hal, **bottom** Roger Job; **139** © Peter Turnley/ CORBIS/MAGMA; **140** © Gilles Saussier/Gamma/PONOPRESSE; **141** © Roger Job/Gamma/PONOPRESSE; **142 top** Sebastian Bolesch/Das Fotoarchiv, **bottom** Tim Dirven/Panos Pictures; **143 top** Tim Dirven/Panos Pictures, **bottom** Jacob Silberberg/Panos Pictures; **144** Tim Dirven/Panos Pictures; **151** Tom Stoddart; **168** Peter Casaer/MSF; **173** Pep Bonet/Panos Pictures; **177** Philippe Desmazes/ AFP/Getty Images; **178** Roger Job; **179** Benno Neeleman; **180** Roger Job; **181** Marleen Daniels/ Hollandse Hoogte; **182** Ton Koene; **183-184** Roger Job; **192** Dan Bortolotti; **198** Jan Banning/Hollandse Hoogte; **203** John Vink/Magnum Photos; **214** AP Photo/Alexander Merkushev; **224** AFP/Getty Images; **249** Ian Berry/ Magnum Photos; **250** Roger Job; **251 top** Roger Job, **bottom** Juan Carlos Tomasi; **252** Sebastian Bolesch/Das Fotoarchiv; **253** Roger Job; **254 top** Roger Job, **bottom** Juan Carlos Tomasi; **255** Carl De Keyser; **256** Ian Berry/Magnum Photos; **267** Eli Reed/Magnum Photos; **Back Cover, top** Carl De Keyser, **bottom** Francesco Zizola/Magnum Photos